OXFORD MEDICAL PUBLICATIONS

Reproductive Medicine: From A to Z

Reproductive Medicine: From A to Z

Editor H. E. Reiss

Principal authors

Mr Peter Brinsden   MB BS, FRCOG
Dr Geraldine Hartshorne   BSc, PhD
Mr Anthony Hirsh   LRCP, MRCS, MB BS, DRCOG, FRCS
Miss Elizabeth Owen   MB BS, MD, MRCOG
Mr Herbert Reiss   MA, BM BCh, FRCOG (Editor)
Rev Dr Michael Reiss   MA, PhD, PGCE, F I Biol

Further contributors

Rev Dr Timothy Appleton   MA, PhD, ScD
Dr Sally C Davies   MB, ChB, MSc, FRCP, MRCPath
Professor Christopher Hudson   MB, MChir, FRCS, FRCOG
Dr Thomas McKee   MB, ChB, PhD, MRCPath
Dr Patricia Munday   MD, FRCOG
Dr Eurof Walters   MA, BSc, PhD

Oxford   New York   Tokyo
OXFORD UNIVERSITY PRESS
1998

Oxford University Press, Great Clarendon Street, Oxford OX2 6DP

Oxford New York
Athens Auckland Bangkok Bogota Bombay
Buenos Aires Calcutta Cape Town Dar es Salaam
Delhi Florence Hong Kong Istanbul Karachi
Kuala Lumpur Madras Madrid Melbourne
Mexico City Nairobi Paris Singapore
Taipei Tokyo Toronto Warsaw

and associated companies in
Berlin Ibadan

Oxford is a trade mark of Oxford University Press

Published in the United States
by Oxford University Press, Inc., New York

A catalogue record for this book is available from the British Library

Library of Congress Cataloging in Publication Data
(Data available)

ISBN 0 19 262901 8

Typeset by Hewer Text Composition Services, Edinburgh

Printed in Great Britain by Biddles Ltd, Guildford, King's Lynn

Acknowledgements

The authors acknowledge with gratitude the inspiration and
help given to them by Professor R.G. Edwards and Dr Eurof
Walters, who first suggested the production of this volume.
A contribution by the International Union of Physiological
Sciences towards expenses is also gratefully acknowledged.

The authors wish to thank the following for kindly granting
permission to reproduce illustrations in this book:

Figures 3 and 6 – Phillips, W.D. and Chilton, T.J. (1994). *A
Level Biology* (revised edition). Oxford University Press.
Figures 2, 7, 10, and 16 – Jeffocoate, T.N.A. *Principles
of Gynaecology* (revised by Tindall, V.R.). Butterworth
Heinemann.
Figure 4 – Roberts, M.B.V, Reiss, M.J, and Monger, G.
Principles and Processes. Thomas Nelson & Sons.
Figures 8 and 27 – Varma, T.R. *Clinical Gynaecology*. Edward
Arnold.
Figure 11 – Garrey, M. *et al.* (1980). *Obstetrics Illustrated.*
(Third edition). Churchill Livingstone.
Figures 14 and 26 – Johnson, M. and Everitt, B.
Essential Reproduction. (Third edition). Blackwell Scientific
Publications.
Figure 21 – Llewellyn-Jones, D. *Fundamentals of Obstetrics
& Gynaecology.*
Figure 24 – *Practical Guide to Reproductive Medicine* (chapter
by Hirsch, A.V.). Parthenon Publications.
Figure 25 – *Concise Medical Dictionary*. Market House.

Foreword

Professor R G Edwards
University of Cambridge

This dictionary is published at a most appropriate time. It coincides with an expansion of knowledge on human reproduction and its associated fields of study. This expansion has been coupled with the introduction of powerful new technologies in science and medicine, including new molecular techniques for diagnosis, micromanipulation, and the immense possibilities inherent in the human genome project. Clinical innovations have kept pace, with advances in endoscopy moving into many new areas of medicine, a deeper awareness of cytokines and other paracrine systems, and the measurement of blood flow by Doppler ultrasound.

Inevitably, these novel approaches to clinical care have resulted in rapid changes in the development of assisted human reproduction. New approaches are promised in ovarian stimulation, to increase efficiency, utilize recombinant hormones and reduce risks to patients, such as hyperstimulation. Male infertility is almost a bygone concept following the introduction of intracytoplasmic injection of a single spermatozoon into an oocyte. Men with very severe infertility due to extreme oligozoospermia can now conceive their own children, by using testicular or epididymal spermatozoa instead of those in the ejaculate, or even spermatids on occasion. At the same time, treatment of men with very few spermatozoa has opened wide aspects of genetics, including highly technical studies on the genetic consequences of microdeletions in Y chromosome DNA. Clinicians have now to relearn about meiosis and chromosome structure, while scientists studying spermatogenesis and oogenesis have to keep up to date with the care of the infertile couple.

Simultaneously, patients are in close touch with many scientific and clinical advances, through the broadcast media, newspapers, and books. They are quickly aware of any new opportunities and their clinical and ethical implications. A new, authoritative dictionary will thus be of immense value to patients and professionals alike, guiding them through the details of contemporary fertility treatment. The dictionary's ethical and counselling entries are highly relevant to patients undergoing complex treatments such as sperm or oocyte donation or surrogacy.

Considerable care and experience was therefore essential in composing the dictionary. Its authors have gone to great lengths to check and verify each entry, and to ensure that the dictionary is easy to use, and well cross-referenced. It has taken them over two years to compile, and they must be delighted at the publication of their carefully prepared texts. Successive sections have been issued on the CD-ROM disc of *Human Reproduction Update*. This gave readers an opportunity to comment on definitions before formal publication of the dictionary. A similar approach will also enable new terms, or modifications, to be added to update the text periodically.

It is a pleasure for me to congratulate Herbert Reiss, who has made immense efforts to coordinate the publication of the dictionary, and Eurof Walters who conceived the original idea. Herbert has worked indefatigably to ensure a smooth flow of information and a series of definitions from his co-authors. All of them have done their best to produce clear, relevant, and up-to-date interpretations within their own specialized fields of study. We must all be grateful to them for their willingness to undertake the task, and complete it on time.

Lastly, I am delighted that Oxford University Press are publishing the dictionary. Their collection of dictionaries is surely second to none. The privilege of having OUP's *Reproductive Medicine: From A to Z* to consult on such personal and clinical matters will undoubtedly add to its authority.

Preface

Infertility has been a cause of unhappiness and despair since the beginnings of humanity. It is referred to in Egyptian Papyri nearly 4000 years old, in the Jewish scriptures, in ancient Chinese medical texts and in the Hippocratic writings. Throughout the ages, afflicted women embraced superstitions and myths about their predicament and resorted to magic and religion for cures. That the male might play a part was rarely considered.

It was not until the Renaissance that Falloppio, in the 16th century, described the anatomy of tube and ovary. A century later van Leeuwenhoek first described the microscopy of spermatozoa and van Graaf that of the ovarian follicle and the seminiferous tubules of the testis. The first recorded and successful case of artificial insemination was documented by John Hunter in 1776. Von Baer described the mammalian egg in 1828 and Marion Sims studied sperm–mucus interaction at the end of the 19th century. Tubal patency tests were introduced in the first half of the present century while reproductive endocrinology and andrology did not become established until its second half.

Throughout this time, treatment of the infertile was in the hands of gynaecologists, latterly with some assistance from endocrinologists and andrologists. The relation of gynaecologist to patient was very personal, one to one, and the infertile woman was unlikely to meet anyone else during her investigations or treatment.

All this has changed radically since the advent of *in vitro* fertilization. The birth of Louise Brown in 1978 not only gave hope to countless couples suffering from what was until then regarded as incurable infertility; it also gave rise to a whole new science of reproductive biology and medicine. Progress arising from the work of Edwards and Steptoe has proceeded at a truly phenomenal pace. Modern management of the subfertile couple has become the province of large multidisciplinary teams. Scientific research is advancing our knowledge of genetics, embryo development, fertilization and implantation. New dimensions are being added to clinical practice on almost a daily basis, involving many other medical specialities. Nurses have a major role in these developments whilst the contributions made by ultrasonographers, counsellors, psychologists, social workers, secretarial staff, administrators and many others are very great.

The processes and issues involved are so profound that they have evoked a multitude of moral and ethical responses. Philosophers, moralists, law makers and politicians, the lay public and those working in the media all now have opinions on the problems of infertility, whilst it remains a truly personal issue for the sufferers.

The terminology employed in the management of these issues has expanded with the growth of the subject. Gynaecologists, scientists and technicians, involved through their work, are often unaware of the precise meaning of terms in daily use. Patients, social scientists, lawyers, ethicists and many others may wish to acquire a closer understanding of terms used. We hope that this volume will help them. To achieve this we have tried to go beyond the bare bones of the definitions and invest them, where appropriate, with explanations and references to clinical relevance.

H.E.R.

Cambridge
July 1997

A

abdominal ostium (*syn.* infundibulum): the fimbriated* end of the Fallopian tube (Fig. 8) and its opening into the abdominal cavity. Occlusion leads to the formation of a hydrosalpinx and is a frequent cause of tubal infertility. (See Fallopian tube, hydrosalpinx.)

abdominal pregnancy: an advanced extra-uterine* pregnancy which has become established in the abdominal cavity and rarely may progress to fetal viability. (See extra-uterine pregnancy.)

abortion: this term comprises spontaneous miscarriage as well as termination of pregnancy. Under UK law, abortion is defined as the expulsion of the fetus/products of conception before the 28th week of pregnancy. Recent advances in neonatal care have led to the survival of a high percentage of births before 28 weeks and the gestational age after which a fetus is considered viable is now generally accepted as 24 weeks. Many clinicians are now defining abortion/miscarriage as the loss of a pregnancy before viability. The World* Health Organization (WHO) definition is 'expulsion or extraction of an embryo or fetus weighing 500 g or less from its mother'. (See miscarriage for clinical details.)

The Abortion Act (1967) legalized termination of pregnancy in the UK under certain clearly defined circumstances. The upper limit for inducing abortions was fixed in the Human Fertilization and Embryology Act* (1990) as 24 weeks with the exception of cases where there is a substantial risk that the baby will be born with serious handicap. The 1967 Act has greatly reduced the morbidity (haemorrhage, sepsis, perforation of uterus) and mortality previously associated with criminal abortion.

abstinence: no sexual activity. In order to standardise sperm* tests, the male partner is usually asked to abstain from intercourse for the preceding three days.

accessory glands of reproduction: in men the glands which manufacture seminal* fluid, primarily the prostate* and seminal* vesicles, but also the bulbo-urethral and peri-urethral glands. (See Fig. 15.)

acid Tyrode solution: the medium* commonly used in embryology to dissolve the zona* pellucida, either by micromanipulation* to make a hole (for sperm entry or assisted* hatching) or completely (as a research tool). It is a mixture of salts of physiological osmolarity, supplemented with glucose, buffered with hydrogen phosphate and titrated to approximately pH 2.5 using hydrochloric acid.

acromegaly (gigantism): a syndrome* which can occur in either sex, caused by secretion of excessive amounts of growth* hormone from an adenoma* of the anterior lobe of the pituitary* gland. In women, this is associated with the development of heavy build, marked enlargement of hands and feet, atrophy of breasts, amenorrhoea* and infertility. Hyperprolactinaemia* is common and there is a risk of diabetes* and cardiovascular disease. Acromegaly is usually self limiting but surgery may be indicated if visual deterioration occurs.

acrosome: the covering (cap) over the anterior two thirds of the head of the spermatozoon* (Fig. 23) which contains the enzymes* involved in the fertilization* process.

acrosome reaction: the process occurring after the spermatozoon* has entered the female genital tract. This leads to the gradual rupture of the acrosome* and the release of enzymes* which enable the sperm to penetrate the cells covering the oocyte* (see cumulus oophorus) and ultimately the final covering of the oocyte, the zona* pellucida*.

activation: cascade of events causing a mature oocyte* to develop beyond its arrest in metaphase* II. Activation normally accompanies fertilization*, but may also occur under artificial conditions not involving spermatozoa* (parthenogenesis*). During fertilization, the oocyte is activated by the penetrating sperm which causes a wave of calcium ion influx, setting in motion the normal events of cortical* granule extrusion, second polar* body extrusion, pronucleus* formation and cytoplasmic* and cytoskeletal changes.

Oocytes can also be activated by artificial stimuli such as a needle prick, incubation in a medium containing calcium ions or ethanol or by electrical pulsing. Artificially activated oocytes may become haploid*, diploid*, polyploid* or mosaic. During cleavage* they may appear identical to normally fertilized embryos, but in humans, their development fails before implantation* because they have no male genetic material (see imprinting).

adenoma: a benign tumour with gland-like structure which grows in glandular tissues such as breast, endocrine glands*, secretory lining of the bowel.

adenomyosis: the presence of endometrium* in an abnormal location in the uterine musculature (myometrium*). Usually adenomyosis is a diffuse infiltrating condition which is not encapsulated; if a single localized area of uterine musculature is affected, this is known as an **adenomyoma**. The aetiology of adenomyosis is unknown: it was formerly called endometriosis interna, but it differs from endometriosis* as it does not spread outside the uterus* and usually (90%) occurs in parous* women. The main symptoms are menorrhagia* and dysmenorrhoea*; the uterus is bulky, irregular and usually tender. Ultrasound* may help in the diagnosis but this is more often made on hysterectomy* specimens from women between the ages of 35 and 50 years.

adhesions: *lit.* from to adhere, become attached, fixed or stuck together. Adhesions can occur anywhere in the body but are commonest between surfaces covered by membranes such as the peritoneum* in the abdomen or the synovial lining in joints. They consist of bands of fibrous tissue, can be vascular or avascular, vary from being velamentous and filmy to dense and rigid and may result in distortion of the anatomy and restricted mobility of organs. They may be caused by trauma, inflammations, endometriosis*, surgery, reaction to foreign bodies or thermal injury.

In the female pelvis, adhesions may interfere with the mobility of the ovaries and tubes upon which ovum* pick-up and transport depend; in the abdomen, interference with motility of the bowel can cause intestinal obstruction; in the uterine* cavity, fibrous bands between endometrial* surfaces can partially or completely obliterate the endometrial cavity (see Asherman's syndrome). Treatment of adhesions is surgical (see adhesiolysis). Prevention of adhesion formation during operations is one of the main objects of modern techniques of microsurgery*.

adhesiolysis: the surgical division of adhesions* to restore normal anatomy and mobility of organs; it is performed by open or laparoscopic* surgery, employing blunt or scalpel dissection, diathermy or laser*.

adhesion molecules: these regulate interactions between cells*, and between cells and matrices. They have a major role in implantation* and possibly also in sperm* binding to the oocyte*.

adnexum: *pl.* adnexa: that which is attached to the uterus, i.e. the Fallopian* tube(s) and ovary(ies)*.

adolescence: the stage of life between childhood and the adult status. Puberty* and, in the female, menarche* occur at this stage.

adoption: the assumption of permanent parental responsibility for a child or children born by another woman who willingly relinquishes responsibility for that child/those children. This differs from fostering which is the temporary placing of a child/children with foster parents. Adoption is often considered as an alternative to assisted reproduction* for childless couples.

In the UK adoption is governed by the Adoption Acts 1958, 1967 and the Children Act 1989 and is regulated by Adoption Societies or Social Services who require assessment and home study reports by social workers, leading to proceedings within the Family Division of the Courts. The various adoption agencies are coordinated by the British Agencies for Adoption and Fostering (BAAF).

Since the Abortion Act (1967) very few babies are available for adoption, resulting in strict criteria for acceptance. Some couples, who are judged to be outside the normal age limits to adopt a baby (35), may be offered an older child, a child with special needs or of mixed race. Inter-country adoption from countries with many homeless children (e.g. Romania, Chile, Thailand) has therefore been considered as an option by some childless couples. Such practice is complicated by different legal and social services procedures between countries.

adrenal glands: two small glands, one situated above each kidney. The adrenal medulla secretes adrenaline and noradrenaline; the cortex secretes mineralocorticoids (e.g. aldosterone), glucocorticoids (e.g. cortisol) and sex hormones (mainly androgens*). Abnormalities of function can lead to adrenogenital* syndrome, Addison's disease, Cushing's* syndrome or phaeochromocytoma.

adrenogenital syndrome (*syn.* congenital adrenal hyperplasia): a rare syndrome* due to a congenital enzyme* defect resulting in decreased cortisol and excess androgen* production. 21 hydroxylase deficiency is the most common form and causes the 'salt losing' type. Chromosomally* normal females may, at birth, have ambiguous external genitalia with marked enlargement of the clitoris* but normal internal genitalia. Treatment is with cortisol; surgery may be required for clitoral reduction. Adult onset adrenogenital syndrome is a milder form with hirsutism*, oligomenorrhoea* or amenorrhoea*.

age: this is also referred to as 'maternal age'; in natural conceptions* in women, fecundity* and fertility* reach their peak by the age of 30. After this fertility declines and spontaneous miscarriage* rates and the incidence of congenital* abnormalities in the offspring rise with increasing age. These changes are more marked in women attempting a first pregnancy, and compounded by heavy smoking. A similar trend is seen in the results of infertility surgery and assisted* reproduction procedures. Ovarian* stimulation and ovum* donation may partially overcome the problem. In men, there is only a slight decline of fertility with increasing age.

agenesis: the absence or failure to develop of a structure, usually as result of a genetic* abnormality. In ovarian agenesis (see Turner's syndrome) the ovaries are rudimentary ('streak') with no germ* cells.

agglutination: the condition where motile spermatozoa* adhere to each other, either head to head (HH), tail to tail (TT) or head to tail (HT); spermatozoa may also adhere to dead sperm, cells or other debris present in the semen*. Agglutination is highly suggestive but not definite proof of the presence of antisperm* antibodies.

AIDS: acquired immunodeficiency syndrome caused by infection by human immunodeficiency virus (HIV)*. This occurs when the immune deficiency caused by HIV is sufficiently severe to cause clinical disease, usually 8 to 10 years after acquiring the infection. The clinical manifestations include infections with organisms which are harmless in healthy individuals (such as *Pneumocystis carinii*) and some tumours such as Kaposi's sarcoma and non-Hodgkin's lymphomas. Altogether there are currently (1997) 28 recognized clinical conditions which constitute a diagnosis of AIDS.

Life expectancy following a diagnosis of AIDS has increased in the years since the syndrome was first recognized in 1981, but survival beyond the third year is unusual. In Western countries, AIDS is much commoner in men than women, but in the developing world where heterosexual transmission of HIV is the normal route of infection, the disease causes high rates of morbidity and mortality in women and children.

AID: artificial insemination using donor sperm. The term has now been replaced by DI (donor insemination) to avoid confusion with AIDS*. (See artificial insemination.)

albumin: a serum protein* (relative molecular mass 69 000) extracted and purified in fractions by electrophoresis. Fraction V is frequently used instead of serum as the protein component of culture* media. Usually human serum albumin (hSA) is used for embryo culture. The functions of albumin in culture medium include limited buffering, the binding of various compounds including steroids* and potentially toxic trace elements and capacitation* of spermatozoa*. Albumin is available as a powder or sterile solution.

albumin gradients: these have been used to separate sperm populations. Claims have been made that separation of spermatozoa* carrying X* (female) and Y* (male) chromosomes is possible. However this method is at best only partially effective and hence not widely accepted.

alcohol abuse: this can have a markedly depressant effect on the quality of semen*. There is also a well recognized fetal* alcohol syndrome, seen in women who have consumed excessive amounts of alcohol in pregnancy.

allele: an alternative form of a gene*. Each of a pair of chromosomes* carries many thousands of genes. In normal (diploid*) cells, genes are found in pairs, one of the pair being inherited from the person's mother, the other from the father. Each gene has its counterpart—allele—on the other chromosome. If the alleles on a pair of chromosomes match, the individual is said to be homozygous* for that gene; if they do not match, heterozygous*.

For example, the cystic* fibrosis gene has a number of alternative alleles, each with its own DNA* sequence. Some of these alleles, so called 'cystic fibrosis alleles', lead to the production of a faulty protein* which can result in cystic fibrosis; so called 'normal alleles' lead to the production of the normal protein.

alpha-feto protein (AFP): an alpha-globulin of similar molecular weight (69 000) to albumin*, synthesized in pregnancy in the yolk* sac and fetal liver. Maternal serum AFP levels rise rapidly in pregnancy as a result of the passage of fetal AFP into the maternal circulation via the placenta*. AFP is present in fetal serum and cerebrospinal fluid at a concentration of about 30 000 times greater than that in maternal serum and 150 times greater than that in amniotic* liquor.

In the presence of open neural* tube defects (see spina bifida, anencephaly), AFP leaks into the amniotic fluid and thus reaches the maternal serum in greater amounts than usual. This raised level of AFP in maternal serum and amniotic fluid is used as a screening* or diagnostic test for open neural tube defects. AFP levels are also raised in multiple* pregnancies, certain other relatively rare congenital* malformations (but not in Down* syndrome) and in cases of intra-uterine death or miscarriage*.

amenorrhoea: absence of menstrual bleeding: this can be primary when menstruation has never occurred (see menarche) or secondary when no menstruation has occurred for more than 3 months in a woman who had a normal menarche. Amenorrhoea is physiological (i.e. normal) before the menarche, during pregnancy or lactation and after the menopause*. Pathological amenorrhoea is not a disease in itself, but a symptom of an underlying abnormality, such as a congenital anomaly, generalized severe illness (e.g. tuberculosis, leukaemia), central nervous system disorder (e.g. certain brain tumours) or nutritional disturbance (anorexia nervosa). Other causes include ovarian disturbances (e.g. polycystic* ovarian disease: the commonest cause of secondary amenorrhoea), other hormonal disturbances (pituitary*, thyroid*), uterine factors (see Asherman's syndrome) and irradiation or chemotherapy.

amino acid: the basic structural unit of proteins*. Amino acids contain amino and carboxyl groups within the same molecule, linked by a central carbon atom and having variable side chains. There are 20 main amino acids; others may be formed by modification of amino acids already incorporated into proteins. They are a source of nitrogen and may be important for some cells in culture.

amnion: the inner of the membranes lining the fetal sac (see also chorion; Fig. 20).

amniotic cavity: the fetal sac containing the embryo*/fetus and the amniotic fluid (liquor). (See Fig. 20.)

amniocentesis: puncture of the amniotic* sac, performed usually early in the second trimester* of pregnancy, in order to withdraw amniotic* fluid and its constituent cells for the antenatal diagnosis of certain congenital* disorders such as neural* tube defects, chromosomal* disorders (see Down's syndrome), and certain metabolic diseases. Since the test provides data on fetal chromosomes, it will also reveal fetal sex. For screening* in pregnancy, this test is used particularly in women over the age of 36 (when there is an increased risk of genetic anomalies) or those with a past history of an affected child.

ampulla: the part of the Fallopian* tube (Figs. 8, 26), between the isthmus* and the infundibulum*; it is approximately 5 cm long, thin walled, wider than the isthmus, and lined internally by large mucosal folds covered by ciliated* epithelium which has a major role in the transport of oocytes*. Fertilization* takes place in the ampulla. It is also a frequent site of extra-uterine* pregnancy and, if the abdominal ostium is occluded, expands to form a hydrosalpinx*.

anabolic steroids: androgenic* drugs, often illegally injected in men wishing to improve athletic performance and increase muscle bulk. As these steroids suppress pituitary gonadotrophins*, the testes* cease sperm production and reduce in size. The man has azoospermia* and the androgens can be metabolized to oestrogens*, leading to breast development.

analysis: method of scientific examination, e.g. semen* analysis.

anaphase: a stage in cell division. Anaphase occurs in both sorts of cell division—meiosis* and mitosis*. It is the stage where the new chromosomes* separate from one another and move to the two different ends of the cell. It is followed by the formation of a new cell membrane between the separated chromosomes, resulting in two new daughter cells.

In mitosis, anaphase begins when the centromeres* split down their middles. This allows each pair of chromatids* to separate into two daughter chromatids, one of which goes to one of the new cells that results from mitosis, the other of which goes to the other. During the first meiotic division homologous chromosomes part company at anaphase (called anaphase I) and move to opposite ends of the cell. In anaphase II, the chromatids part company and move to opposite ends of the cell.

Anaphase is over within a matter of minutes. However, mistakes during anaphase I or anaphase II in meiosis can have profound, long-term consequences, because they may lead to daughter cells having differing numbers of chromosomes. This is known as non-disjunction*. The most important chromosome mutation resulting from non-disjunction is the one that causes Down's syndrome*, in which an affected individual has 47 rather than 46 chromosomes in each cell.

anastomosis: in surgery, the connection made, usually by stitching, between the two separated ends of a tubular structure: e.g. of the Fallopian* tube or vas* deferens (vaso-vasostomy*) after occlusion or division by a sterilization operation. Similarly in males an epididymo-vasostomy* is carried out to by-pass an epididymal obstruction and in women an obstruction at the utero-tubal* junction may be excised with anastomosis of the healthy cut ends.

androgens: steroid* hormones* (e.g. testosterone*, androstenedione) produced by the testes*, adrenal* cortex and, in small amounts, the ovaries*. In the male, androgens are concerned with development and maintenance of the secondary sexual* characteristics; in the female they are precursors for oestrogen* production. If there is excessive secretion in women, defeminization (amenorrhoea*, breast atrophy) and masculinizing changes (male hair distribution, deep voice, enlarged clitoris*) may result. (See hyperandrogenism.)

andrology: the medical speciality concerned with fertility and sexual disorders in men. (See semen analysis, CASA, antisperm antibodies, acrosome reaction, azoospermia, vas deferens obstruction, varicocele, premature ejaculation, impotence.)

anejaculation: failure to ejaculate. (See aspermia, spinal injury.)

anembryonic pregnancy: a pregnancy where an empty gestational* sac and rudimentary placenta* are present, but no fetus has formed: this is usually noted by ultrasound* scanning and leads to an inevitable or missed miscarriage*. (See also biochemical pregnancy, blighted ovum.)

anencephaly: an embryological defect of the neural* tube, with absence of the vault of the skull, gross malformation of the brain, and usually associated with spina* bifida. Anencephaly results in stillbirth or early neonatal* death; it can be diagnosed antenatally by ultrasound* or X-rays, and also by raised alpha-feto* protein levels in maternal blood and amniotic* liquor.

aneuploidy: the loss or gain of one or two chromosomes*. In a healthy human, all the cells except the germ cells (oocyte and sperm) have 46 chromosomes. However during the formation of the germ cells or around the time of fertilization*, mistakes sometimes occur which result in each cell having e.g. 44, 45, 47 or 48 chromosomes.

An embryo with only 44 or fewer chromosomes never survives the whole pregnancy and is lost by spontaneous miscarriage. Most embryos with 45, 47 or 48 chromosomes also perish, but some examples of aneuploidy do result in live births: the best known and most frequent is Down's* syndrome. Other examples are Turner's* and Klinefelter's* syndromes or XYY disorders.

anorchism: a rare disorder where a man has no testes*; this is usually the result of disease or injury, but can be due to degeneration in early uterine life. Patients are deficient in androgens* and therefore eunuchoidal (immature). They cannot be made fertile and require androgen* therapy to assist with sexual function. Anorchism must not be confused with cryptorchism*, where the testes have failed to descend and there is better virilization, but also an increased risk of testicular tumours.

anorexia nervosa: a nutritional disorder, psycho-somatic in origin and characterized by loss of appetite, leading to severe weight loss, emaciation and, if not treated, death. Secondary amenorrhoea* and anovulation* usually occur and are associated with low FSH* and LH* concentrations.

anorgasmia: failure to achieve orgasm* (climax) during sexual intercourse.

anosmia: absence of sense of smell. (See Kallmann's syndrome.)

anovulation: absence of ovulation*. Anovulatory cycles are menstrual cycles without ovulation* and corpus* luteum formation; they tend to be irregular cycles, sometimes shorter, often longer, than normal.

anteversion: the normal position of the uterus* in the body with forward inclination of the cervix* and uterus at an angle of about 90 degrees to the axis of the vagina*. (See retroversion.)

antibody: also called immunoglobulin: a group of proteins* synthesized in response to a foreign substance, known as antigen. The antibody is specific for the antigen and will bind to it as part of the immune response (see immunity). The various types of antibody are classified according to their structure, IgA, IgD, IgE, IgG, IgM and play different roles in the immune response.

Infertility may occur when antibodies form against spermatozoa (see antisperm antibodies) and circulate in the woman's body, or are present in the cervical* mucus, binding to sperm cells and interfering with their normal function. Antisperm antibodies may be found in the serum of either partner, and/or in seminal* plasma.

Another example is the Rhesus antibody, raised in response to isoimmunization of a Rhesus negative woman from a Rhesus positive fetus. (See haemolytic disease of the new-born.)

antibody screening: this is routinely performed on maternal serum at the first antenatal booking and, again, at 28 weeks of pregnancy to exclude the presence of atypical antibodies* that could give rise to haemolytic* disease of the newborn. Rh(D) negative women generally have a third antibody check at 32–34 weeks gestation. (See screening.)

antigen: see antibody.

anti-oestrogen: a drug which attenuates the effect of oestrogen* in the body. Clomiphene* is such a drug and may be successful in the treatment of infertility when used to stimulate and regulate oocyte* production. It has been used to try and stimulate spermatogenesis* in the male, but with little success. (See also Tamoxifen.)

antisperm antibodies: these may be found in the serum of either partner, as well as in cervical* mucus in the female and seminal* plasma in the male; they lead to immunological* infertility by coating the spermatozoa and interfering with normal sperm function. In women sperm cells are 'foreign' and may therefore be recognized by the immune system. Sperm antibodies are detected on spermatozoa by the mixed agglutination reaction (MAR)* or immunobead* tests; they can be found in the serum of either partner by the Kibrick, tray agglutination (TAT*) and immunobead* tests.
   Antibodies may bind only to specific regions of the sperm, e.g. head, tail or mid-piece. They cause spermatozoa to stick together (see agglutination), thereby reducing their motility. However even apparently normal motile sperm may be coated and thereby hindered in their passage through cervical* mucus and in their fertilizing ability. In men, the blood–testis barrier normally protects spermatozoa from auto-immune attack, but serum antibodies may form if the barrier is damaged (e.g. by trauma or surgery such as vasectomy*). Treatment of antisperm antibodies may be attempted with steroids* to suppress the immune response, but this therapy is by no means always successful and carries risks from side effects. IVF* is now more often employed in treatment. (See antibody.)

antrum: the central cavity inside a developing ovarian follicle* (Fig. 6), filled with follicular* fluid. It expands as the follicle grows, to occupy most of its volume shortly before ovulation*.

Apgar score: a method of assessing the condition of the new-born infant, at one and five minutes after delivery, based on observations of the heart rate, respiratory effort, muscle tone, response to stimuli and skin colour. It is named after Virginia Apgar, American paediatrician.

aplasia: incomplete development of an organ. In women, ovarian aplasia is a synonym for Turner's* syndrome. In men vas* deferens aplasia (congenital absence of the vas deferens) is an important cause of azoospermia*.

appendicitis: inflammation of the appendix. If perforation occurs, this may lead to pelvic peritonitis and subsequent tubal infertility.

artery: blood vessel carrying blood from the heart to all parts of the body, including the internal organs.

ARIC: (acrosome reaction with ionophore challenge): a diagnostic laboratory test of the adequacy of the acrosome* reaction of spermatozoa*, and therefore their ability to fertilize.

artificial insemination: the introduction of semen* into the female genital tract by means other than sexual intercourse. Deposition of semen can be in the vagina*, cervical* canal or uterus* (intra-uterine* insemination: IUI).
   Artificial insemination with the husband's semen (AIH) is used mainly in patients with psychosexual problems (impotence*, premature ejaculation*) or, by IUI, to bypass an unfavourable cervix* or treat immunological* or unexplained* infertility. Donor insemination* (DI) is used in cases with absolute male infertility (e.g. Klinefelter's* syndrome; hypogonadism*) or in treatment-resistant azoospermia* and other sperm defects. Nowadays only frozen semen is used in DI to guard against accidental transmission of HIV*. (See HIV, AIDS and donor insemination.)

Use of the term AID (artificial insemination donor) has been abandoned in favour of DI to avoid confusion.

artificial spermatocele: a surgically constructed reservoir for spermatozoa* in cases of irreversible obstructive* azoospermia or ejaculation* failure. Spermatozoa are aspirated from the reservoir for use in assisted conception. The use of such reservoirs is now being discontinued in view of advances with intra-cytoplasmic* injection of spermatozoa obtained by new techniques of testicular* or epididymal* aspiration (Fig. 24).

Asherman's syndrome: the partial or complete obliteration of the uterine* cavity by adhesions* (synechiae) caused by endometrial* infection or over-vigorous curettage* after miscarriage* or childbirth; depending on the extent and severity of the adhesions, spontaneous miscarriage*, amenorrhoea* or infertility* may occur.

Aschheim–Zondek test: the first biological pregnancy test. The presence of chorionic* gonadotrophins in urine, when injected into immature female mice, resulted in ovarian changes indicative of pregnancy. Other biological pregnancy tests were performed on rabbits (Friedman test), rats and male toads (*xenopus*). All are now superseded by immunological pregnancy* tests.

ascites: the accumulation of fluid in the peritoneal cavity which can be caused by many conditions such as heart failure, liver disease and tumours (especially ovarian). Ascites also occurs in severe cases of ovarian* hyperstimulation syndrome (OHSS).

aspermatogenesis: no sperm production in the testes*. This may be total (azoospermia*) or partial (oligozoospermia*). Causes of aspermatogenesis include trauma to the testes, infection (e.g. bilateral mumps* orchitis*), torsion, untreated undescended* testes (cryptorchism), genetic disorders (e.g. Klinefelter's* syndrome) and irradiation.

aspermia: failure to discharge seminal* fluid at orgasm*. This failure of ejaculation* must not be confused with azoospermia* when there are no spermatozoa in the seminal fluid or with retrograde* ejaculation when semen is discharged into the bladder.

assay: a system by which a substance can be quantified accurately by comparison with known standard amounts of the same substance. All assays exploit some special characteristic of the substance under investigation which will permit its detection, such as enzymatic* activity, structure (to which an antibody* may bind) or bioactivity. Assays vary in their sensitivity* and specificity* depending on the exact mechanism by which they work. For this reason, different assays of the same substance may not give identical results. In reproductive medicine, assays are often used to measure levels of hormones* in blood or urine.

assisted fertilization (Fig. 1): micro-manipulation* designed to promote the chance of fertilization* *in vitro*, usually when fertilization has failed previously, or when the quality of the semen* is too poor to allow routine IVF* insemination methods.

Fertilization may fail because of various factors affecting either spermatozoa* or oocytes* or both: these factors include very low sperm concentration, motility or progression*; absence of complementary receptors; inability of spermatozoa to undergo capacitation* or acrosome* reaction;

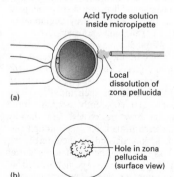

Fig. **1**. Assisted Fertilisation
Fig. **1.1**. Zona drilling (ZD).

a. Acid released locally against the zona pellucida dissolves it away, leaving a hole through which sperm can enter the oocyte.
b. Surface view of the hole formed.

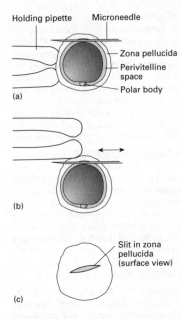

(a)
- Zona pellucida
- Perivitelline space
- Polar body

Holding pipette   Microneedle

(b)

(c)   Slit in zona pellucida (surface view)

Fig. **1.2**. Partial zona dissection (PZD).
a. Solid microneedle is inserted through the zona pellucida of a mature oocyte secured on a holding pipette.
b. The oocyte is released from the holding pipette and the area of zone pellucida trapped by the microneedle is rubbed against the holding pipette until it has been abraded to form a slit.
c. Surface view of slit formed in the zona pellucida, through which sperm can enter the oocyte.

sperm immaturity; an unusually tough or thick zona* pellucida and unknown conditions where both oocytes and spermatozoa appear to be normal.
   The following techniques of assisted fertilization are used:

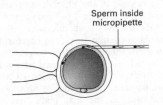

Fig. **1.3**. Subzonal insertion (SUZI). Sperm are loaded into a hollow needle. The needle is inserted under the zona pellucida of an oocyte and one or more sperm are allowed to swim out into the perivitelline space.

Sperm inside micropipette

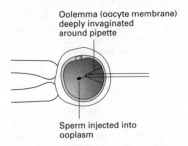

Oolemma (oocyte membrane) deeply invaginated around pipette

Sperm injected into ooplasm

Fig. **1.4**. Intracytoplasmic sperm injection (ICSI). A single sperm is immobilised and injected through the zona pellucida and directly into the cytoplasm of the oocyte.

(1) Zona drilling: the chemical dissolution of part of the zona* pellucida to form a hole through which spermatozoa can enter.

(2) Partial zona dissection (PZD), also called zona slitting: the mechanical cutting of the zona pellucida using a microscopic glass needle, to make a slit through which spermatozoa can enter.

(3) Sub-zonal insertion (SUZI): injection of one or more living spermatozoa underneath the zona pellucida and next to the oocyte surface.

(4) Intra-cytoplasmic* sperm injection (ICSI): injection of a single spermatozoon through the oocyte membrane (see oolemma) and into the oocyte itself. This is the most successful method developed to date and may achieve fertilization rates in excess of 50%.

assisted hatching (AH): the mechanical or chemical breaching of the zona* pellucida using micro-manipulation* to provide a hole through which the blastocyst* can escape (hatch). AH is usually performed on embryos in early cleavage*. Its use may be indicated when the zona pellucida is particularly thick or tough, when implantation* has failed despite repeated transfers of apparently good quality embryos, or when a small hole is already present in which the hatching embryo could become stuck.

assisted reproductive technology (ART): that part of reproductive medicine which deals with means of conception* other than normal coitus*. ART frequently involves the handling of gametes* or embryos*, and includes one or more of the following: ovarian* stimulation; oocyte* collection; sperm* preparation; *in vitro* fertilization (IVF); embryo* transfer (ET); intra-uterine* insemination (IUI); donor* insemination (DI); micro manipulation*, e.g. subzonal* injection (SUZI) and intracytoplasmic* sperm injection (ICSI); gamete intrafallopian transfer (GIFT*); pronucleate* stage tubal transfer (PROST); cryopreservation* and other related procedures.

Those procedures which involve the handling of embryos or donated gametes* are controlled by the Human* Fertilisation and Embryology Authority (HFEA).

association: a statistical term with a meaning similar to correlation* but more usually used for the interdependance of discrete* variables, such as the presence or absence of two diseases in individuals. Such data could be displayed in a 2 by 2 contingency* table, and a measure of association, of which several have been proposed in the literature, used to quantify the interdependence of the two diseases.

asthenospermia: see the correct term, asthenozoospermia.

asthenozoospermia: reduced sperm motility. By definition, this is diagnosed when less than 50% of spermatozoa have forward movement or less than 25% have rapid movement.

atresia: absence, imperforation or closure of a normal opening. This may apply to canalized structures such as the vagina or cervical canal, or to ovarian follicles which, having never fully matured, degenerate without having ruptured to release an ovum.

atrophy: degeneration after development: e.g. testicular atrophy after torsion.

autoimmune disease: a disease resulting from the reaction of one or more components of the immune system with a constituent of the inivdual's own body (self antigen). This is thought to result from a breakdown of tolerance, the process by which the immune system is de-sensitized to self antigens. Immunological tolerance can be broken in various ways including release of self antigens previously inaccessible to the immune system (e.g. the formation of antisperm* antibodies following trauma or surgery) or following infection by microorganisms that can mimic self antigens. The inflammatory reaction set up by this aberrant immune response can result in premature* ovarian failure and early* pregnancy loss.

autosomal disorder: a genetic abnormality in which the fault lies with one or more of the 44 autosomes* rather than with one or both of the sex chromosomes*. The significance of this is that males and females are equally likely to suffer from autosomal disorders, and therefore equally likely to pass them on to their children. Cystic fibrosis* and sickle-cell anaemia* are examples of autosomal disorders.

autosome: in humans, one of the 44 non-sex chromosomes*. The only chromosomes that are not autosomes are the X* and Y* chromosomes.

average: in common usage, the word average generally refers to the arithmetic mean value. As a measure of location, it has some competitors (mode, median) but the average is the most widely used statistic, the easiest to compute, and perhaps the most widely understood measure of location. These three measures of location coincide for symmetrical distributions.

azoospermia: absence of spermatozoa* in the semen*. This may be due to failure of sperm production in the testes*, often called secretory azoospermia (in which case the serum FSH* concentration is raised) , or to a blockage in the efferent duct systems, called obstructive* azoospermia. In the secretory form, micro-aspiration methods are now frequently successful in recovering very small numbers of spermatozoa which are used for intracytoplasmic* sperm injection (ICSI), whilst cases of obstructive azoospermia are, in the first place, treated surgically (see epididymo-vasostomy).

A variety of chromosomal* abnormalities are found in up to 20% of men with impaired spermatogenesis*: the incidence is lower in men with low sperm counts and higher in those with azoospermia. For this reason men with azoospermia or severe oligozoospermia* should have appropriate genetic* counselling before commencing treatment with ICSI*. Azoospermia must not be confused with aspermia* where there is no semen.

B

Bacterial vaginosis (BV): this condition, also known as non-specific vaginitis, Gardnerella vaginitis and anaerobic vaginosis, is the commonest cause of vaginal discharge in sexually active women. The discharge is grey with a fishy odour. True itching does not occur but there may be vulval* soreness. *Gardnerella vaginalis* is only one of many micro-organisms, normally found in the vagina, whose numbers increase enormously to produce the characteristic clinical findings. Diagnosis is made clinically (typical discharge, raised vaginal pH, presence of 'clue cells' and positive amine test) or on examination of a stained vaginal smear. Treatment is with oral metronidazole or clindamycin vaginal cream. Recent data suggest that BV is associated with both pelvic* inflammatory disease and pre-term delivery.

bacterium: *pl.* bacteria. Single-celled organisms which usually reproduce rapidly by cell division, but may remain dormant as spores. They have a simpler organization than animal or plant cells and are widely distributed in soil (where they have a role in the decomposition of dead organic matter), as well as in water and living organisms. Pathogenic bacteria are those which produce diseases (e.g. in humans, cholera, tuberculosis, gonorrhoea, diphtheria). Bacterial infections can be treated by antibiotics such as penicillin or streptomycin, but the evolution of antibiotic-resistant strains is a serious problem.

Banding: Chromosomes* can be stained in a number of different ways to reveal alternating patches of dark and light, called bands. These bands are characteristic of a particular chromosome and so make it possible to distinguish chromosomes that are very similar in length and shape, such as chromosomes 10 and 11.

Barr body: a densely staining area, consisting of sex chromatin*, present in the nucleus* in about 50% of female cells. In women each cell contains two X chromosomes*, but the cell uses only one of them. The other chromosome, which is partially inactive, forms a small dense mass, the Barr body. Presence or absence of the Barr body has been used in the diagnosis of genetic sex, e.g. babies born with ambiguous external genitalia, in the diagnosis of azoospermic* men with Klinefelter's* syndrome and also in athletes of masculine appearance, claiming to be female. Newer techniques for the diagnosis of genetic sex are now available and so the Barr body method is less frequently used.

Bartholin's gland: the pea-sized, mucus secreting gland situated in the lower part of each labium* majus and connected by a duct to the vaginal entrance; its secretion contributes to vaginal lubrication. Inflammation may lead to abscess formation, whilst obstruction of the duct causes a Bartholin gland cyst.

basal body temperature (BBT): ovulation* leads to increased blood progesterone* concentrations which are associated with a small rise in body temperature. Daily recordings of the temperature under standard conditions (before rising in the morning, and before eating or drinking) show a lower temperature during menstruation and in the follicular* phase of the cycle, with a post-ovulatory rise, in the secretory* phase, of approximately 0.5 °C. The woman also marks on the chart the days when intercourse has occurred.

A typical 'biphasic' (Fig. 2) chart usually indicates that ovulation has occurred, but other charts can be difficult to interpret. The temperature remains elevated if pregnancy has occurred.

beta-thalassaemia: a hereditary blood disorder (see haemoglobinopathy). When a person has only one β-thalassaemia gene*, they are known as β-thalassaemia carriers (trait) and they may have a mild anaemia associated with abnormally small red blood

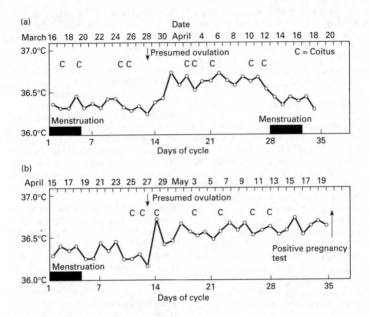

Fig. 2. Basal Body Temperature. The biphasic temperature chart typical of a menstrual cycle (a) in which ovulation has occurred, and (b) in which conception has taken place.

cells (microcytosis). Those with two abnormal genes, one inherited from each parent, suffer from a serious blood disorder and require repeated treatment with blood transfusions. The β-thalassaemia trait occurs only rarely in North Europeans and is most common in people of Mediterranean, Arab and sub-Saharan origin. The trait can be detected by screening*: when both parents are carriers, counselling and ante-natal diagnosis are available.

bicornuate uterus: uterus divided into two, usually equal sized, compartments (Fig. 16) due to failure of complete fusion of the two Müllerian ducts* during embryonic development. The diagnosis is made by hysterosalpingography*, ultrasound* or hysteroscopy*. A bicornuate uterus can be associated with menorrhagia*, recurrent* miscarriages, malpresentation of the fetus and other obstetric problems. Surgical correction is only very occasionally indicated.

binovular twins: see dizygotic twins, multiple pregnancy.

biochemical pregnancy (pre-clinical abortion/miscarriage): a failed pregnancy, diagnosed by a rise and subsequent fall in the serum concentration of human* chorionic gonadotrophin; there is failure of implantation* or early embryonic death and no embryo is detected on ultrasound* scanning. Menstruation may not be delayed, or may be postponed by only a few days and the conceptus is lost with the menstrual flow. This sequence of events probably happens very often without the woman's knowledge. In IVF*, pregnancies are diagnosed very early by raised βhCG concentrations and therefore most 'biochemical' pregnancies are found in this context. (See also anembryonic pregnancy, blighted ovum.)

biopsy: the taking of a small piece of tissue from a living (or dead) subject for laboratory examination. Cervical* tissue and uterine endometrium* are frequently biopsied in the diagnosis of disease or hormonal status. Chorionic* villus sampling and pre-implantation embryo biopsy are used for the prenatal detection of certain congenital* abnormalities (see pre-implantation diagnosis). Testicular* biopsy is employed to diagnose the cause of azoospermia* in infertile men and is now also performed to obtain spermatozoa* for ICSI* (see testicular sperm extraction).

birth rates: see live birth rates.

birthweight: The average weight of a new-born infant is about 3 kg (approximately 7½ lbs). There are large variations associated with genetic, ethnic and environmental (e.g. maternal nutrition) factors. Low birthweight can be the result of prematurity, intrauterine growth retardation or multiple* pregnancy. All these three factors may be operative in babies conceived by IVF* and some other forms of ART*. Very low birth weight, associated with prematurity, is the commonest cause of neonatal mortality* and may be associated with various degrees of mental or physical impairment in the survivors.

blastocoele: the fluid-filled cavity of the blastocyst*. In humans, the blastocoele forms on about day 4 or 5 when the compacted* embryo forms tight junctions between the cells around its periphery. These outer cells (nascent trophectoderm*) begin to pump fluid into the extra-cellular space inside the embryo. The fluid has no connection with the external environment of the embryo and forms an embryo-conditioned micro-environment in which the inner cell mass* and mesoderm develop.

blastocyst (Fig. 7): the stage at which the embryonic cells have differentiated into trophectoderm* and inner* cell mass layers, with formation of a blastocoelic* cavity. The trophectoderm will form the placenta* and fetal membranes; the fetus will develop from the inner cell mass. In humans, blastocyst formation occurs about day 5 of development. At this stage the blastocyst contains about 100 cells and is still contained within the zona* pellucida, although cell division is continuing. Expansion of the blastocoele increases the embryo's volume and stretches the zona pellucida. The embryo must escape from the zona pellucida before implantation* can occur on about day 7. *In vitro*, embryos 'hatch' through a breach in the zona, but it is not known whether the same occurs *in vivo*.

blastomere: an individual cell of an embryo. This term is usually applied to cells in cleavage* stage embryos.

blighted ovum: non-viable pregnancy where an empty gestational* sac is detected by ultrasound*. The fetus is absent or rudimentary. This is usually the result of a genetic* abnormality. (See also anembryonic pregnancy, biochemical pregnancy.)

blood groups: there are inherited biochemical differences on the surface of red blood cells that can act as antigens* and raise antibody* responses if transfused into antigen negative people. This can then lead to red cell destruction (haemolysis). The main blood group systems are ABO, Rhesus and Kell; altogether there are up to 100 other blood group systems with major and minor alleles* that can give rise to immunization and, consequently, problems at crossmatching* of blood.

Patients should always be given ABO compatible blood, otherwise a life-threatening haemolytic transfusion reaction can occur. Women of childbearing age (and girls) should be given Rh(D) compatible blood in order to ensure that they are not immunized. (See also haemolytic disease of the new-born.)

blood pressure: term used to describe the pressure in blood vessels produced by the pumping action of the heart against the peripheral resistance of the arteries. The blood pressure thus varies with the efficiency of cardiac action, the elasticity of the arteries, the volume and viscosity of the blood and the size of the vascular bed. A satisfactory blood pressure is essential to maintain the circulation and supply of blood to individual organs. Blood pressure is measured in millimetres of mercury (mmHg).

The blood pressure may vary with many factors, including the age, height and weight of an individual. Diseases of the heart, kidneys and arteries can cause significant variations from the normal. In pregnancy a raised blood pressure may be associated with reduced blood flow to the uterus* and interfere with placental* function and fetal growth; it can also predispose to the development of pre-eclampsia*.

Some drugs, such as thiazide diuretics and beta-blockers, used to lower raised blood pressure in men, can produce impotence*.

Braxton Hicks contractions: painless, intermittent contractions of the uterus* in pregnancy which do not cause dilatation of the cervix*.

breech: lower pole of the fetus. In breech presentation this is the part of the fetus which enters the birth canal first.

broad ligaments: bilateral folds of peritoneum* which stretch from the sides of the uterus* to the pelvic walls and enclose blood vessels, lymphatics and nerves that supply the uterus (Fig. 8). The Fallopian* tubes are enclosed in the upper border of each broad ligament.

bromocriptine: brand name Parlodel; a drug which belongs to the group known as dopamine* agonists, used in the treatment of hyperprolactinaemia* to restore menstruation* and ovulation*.

buserelin: brand names Suprecur and Suprefact: a drug which belongs to the group known as gonadotrophin* releasing hormone (GnRH) analogues, used to desensitize the pituitary* gland and decrease the output of FSH* and LH*; this causes the ovaries* to become quiescent and subsequently respond to stimulation* in a more predictable manner.

C

Caesarean section: the surgical operation to deliver the fetus and placenta by incising the abdominal wall and usually the lower segment of the uterus*; anaesthesia (general or regional) is required; the operation can be performed before the onset of labour (elective), or during labour (emergency) if unexpected fetal or maternal problems have arisen.

Candida albicans: a fungus which infects skin and mucous membranes of the oral cavity and ano-genital region, causing the condition known as thrush (candidiasis, monilia, yeast infection). The organism is a normal inhabitant of the genital and lower alimentary tracts, and only causes the typical symptoms of itching and a thick, curdy white discharge, when rapid multiplication occurs with the appearance of the active form of the fungus (mycelium). Predisposing factors include the use of antibiotics and steroids*, diabetes mellitus* and local trauma. *C. albicans* may infect men and may be transmitted sexually. In men, an inflammation of the glans penis* and foreskin occurs with a rash. Diagnosis is made by microscopy and culture, and treatment with a wide range of local and orally active agents is available. The partner should be treated simultaneously. Some women suffer frequent recurrences and require specialist investigation.

capacitation: the final phase of development of spermatozoa* when they acquire the ablity to fertilize* an oocyte*. Although previously considered to occur after ejaculation* when the spermatozoa have left the seminal* plasma in the vagina and entered the upper female reproductive tract, capacitation clearly occurs in the laboratory in order that in-vitro* fertilization (IVF) can take place. Scientists therefore question the nature of capacitation. The process takes about 4 to 6 hours and is marked by the development of hyperactivated (erratic) sperm motility, prior to the acrosome* reaction and fusion with the zona* pellucida of the oocyte.

carbon dioxide (CO_2): a gas which is a by-product of respiration. Concentrations in air are approximately 0.04%, but concentrations in the body tissues are 5%. For this reason, most culture* media contain bicarbonate ions and cells are cultured in a CO_2 rich atmosphere to provide appropriate physiological conditions. CO_2 is also used for the induction of the pneumoperitoneum* which precedes laparoscopy*.

carcinoma-in-situ: the earliest, noninvasive stage of cancer. In the cervix it is known as cervical* intra-epithelial neoplasia (CIN) and diagnosed by the performance of Pap* smears. (See cervical smear.) Carcinoma-in-situ is also found in the vulva* when it is known as vulval intra-epithelial neoplasia and occasionally in the testis* when it can lead to testicular cancer. The risk is increased in undescended* testes.

cardinal ligaments: also known as transverse cervical or Mackenrodt's ligaments; fibrous bands of tissue extending from the sides of the lower cervix* and upper vagina* to the lateral pelvic walls, thus forming the central part of the pelvic floor and supporting the uterus* and vaginal vault.

CASA (computer assisted semen analysis): an automated method of carrying out semen* analysis with the ability to study sperm motion and define characteristics such as lateral head displacement (LHD), hyperactivated motility, straight line (progressive) velocity (VSL), curvilinear velocity (VCL) and mean path velocity (VAP). Some of these indices have been linked to sperm fertilizing ability, but CASA is used primarily for research.

castration: the removal of the ovaries* or testes*. This has been used clinically in the treatment of breast or prostatic* cancer. The term must not be confused with sterilization*.

cell (Fig. 3): the basic building block of life. In mammals, it comprises a

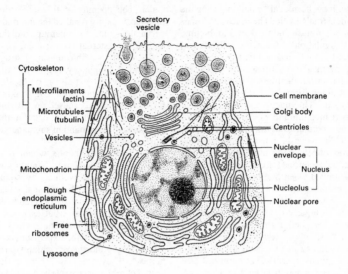

Fig. 3. Cell. Generalised human cell showing structures revealed by electron microscopy.

membrane-bound collection of organelles, contains a nucleus* (except red blood cells and platelets) and is capable of producing and responding to biological stimuli. Cells are extremely diverse in shape, size and function. Examples of cells include oocytes*, spermatozoa*, blastomeres*, neurons.

centromere: the point at which the two chromatids* of a chromosome* are joined. Some chromosomes have their centromere at their middle; others have it nearer one end (see karyotype).

cervical incompetence: a condition of the cervix associated with some cases of recurrent* miscarriage. The internal* cervical os is patulous (open), so that the enlarging fetal sac is no longer adequately retained in the uterine cavity and herniates into the vagina.

Clinically the diagnosis is made from the typical history of repeated, painless, second trimester* miscarriages, usually starting with rupture of the membranes and resulting rapidly in the virtually painless expulsion of a normal fetus. There may also be a history of repeated premature onset of labour, starting with spontaneous rupture of the membranes. The diagnosis can be confirmed by the ready acceptance by the non-pregnant cervix of a size

8 Hegar dilator or by hysterosalpingographic* or ultrasound* evaluation of the cervical canal.

Cervical incompetence can be caused by excessive dilatation* of the cervix, obstetric trauma or be associated with an infantile (hypoplastic) type of uterus. Treatment in the non-pregnant state has been abandoned in favour of a 'cerclage' type of operation to narrow the lumen of the cervical canal, performed towards the end of the first trimester* and after confirmation of an otherwise normal pregancy. (See Shirodkar operation.)

cervical intra-epithelial neoplasia (CIN): this is a change in the cells* of the cervix* which is asymptomatic, usually detected by abnormal cervical* smears and confirmed by colposcopy* and/or biopsy*. Some lesions regress spontaneously, others may become invasive, often after many years. This is preventable by treatment with excision, diathermy coagulation, laser* vaporization or cryosurgery* of the cervix. (See also carcinoma-in-situ, cervical smear.)

cervical mucus: the secretion from the glandular epithelium* lining the cervical* canal: its quantity, quality, viscosity (known as Spinnbarkeit*) and crystallization (known as ferning*) vary with the hormonal* changes during the menstrual* cycle. The mucus becomes more profuse and fluid around the time of ovulation* (under the influence of oestradiol*) and at this time is easily penetrated by spermatozoa* which survive in its alkaline environment after escaping from the acidity of the upper vagina. The mucus acts both as transport medium and as storage depot for the spermatozoa. In the second half of the cycle the mucus becomes thick and impenetrable under the influence of progesterone* (a change deliberately achieved when oral contraceptives are administered).

Deficient amounts of mucus, failure to liquefy or excessive cellularity may be noted during the performance of post-coital* tests and can be important causes of subfertility. A cervical mucus–sperm penetration test (see Kremer penetration test) may be performed in cases of negative or abnormal post-coital tests. Bovine cervical mucus can be used for carrying out this test instead of human cervical mucus. The cervical mucus can also contain agglutinating and immobilizing anti-sperm* antibodies which interfere with sperm motility (cervical hostility) and prevent their ascent into the upper genital tract.

cervical smear (Papanicolaou or Pap* smear): these smears consist of cells* scraped by means of a specially shaped wooden or plastic spatula from the the transformation (transitional) zone of the external* cervical os. The cells thus obtained are stained and examined microscopically (cytology) to detect pre-cancerous changes (see cervical intra-epithelial carcinoma). Lower genital tract infections can also be diagnosed during cytological examinations. Screening* women by means of cervical smears is one of the great advances in preventive medicine and, provided the uptake is high enough and screening is repeated at regular intervals, the incidence of cervical cancer can be greatly reduced. In the UK the recommended interval between Pap tests for women who have never had an abnormal smear is 3 years.

cervix (Fig. 26): the lower part of the uterus*, which projects into the upper vagina* and is traversed by the cervical canal. The opening of the canal into the uterine cavity is called the internal* cervical os, and the opening into the vagina, the external* cervical os.

The cervix is a fibro-muscular structure and, in pregnancy, acts as a bottle neck to prevent expulsion of the fetus. Dilatation and shortening ('taking up') of the canal, caused by uterine contraction and retraction, occur in the first stage of labour and in spontaneous miscarriages.

The part of the cervix which projects into the vagina is known as the exocervix and is lined by squamous epithelium*; the cervical canal above this is lined by a glandular epthelium. Both these, but especially the endocervical epithelium, are highly sensitive to acute infections (acute cervicitis) e.g. gonorrhoea*, chlamydia*, herpes*. They may also become the seat of chronic cervicitis. The glandular epithelium of the endocervical canal is under the control of the ovarian hormones*. In its lower reaches, there are crypts which act as depots for the storage of spermatozoa and where the cervical* mucus, which plays an essential role in sperm transit through the cervical canal, is produced.

A cervical erosion is the extension of the glandular epithelium from the canal onto the exocervix: this is caused by hormonal changes and requires no treatment. Tears of the cervix following childbirth or over-vigorous dilatation may cause ectropion* of the external os. Overstretching of the internal os may lead to cervical* incompetence and cause recurrent* second trimester* miscarriages. The zone where squamous and glandular epithelium meet is known as the transformation (transition) zone and is a frequent site of abnormal cell changes, detected by cervical* smears, some of which may ultimately become malignant (cancerous) if not treated (see cervical intra-epithelial carcinoma). Treatment of chronic cervicitis or pre-malignant changes (diagnosed by cytology smears) may be by excision of a cervical cone, by diathermy coagulation, laser* vaporization or by cryosurgery*.

chiasma (*pl.* chiasmata): the point at which two chromatids* break at the same place and then exchange their genetic* material before the breaks are mended. The formation of chiasmata is known as 'crossing-over' and is perfectly normal. Its importance in evolution is that it allows genes to be swapped between maternal and paternal chromosomes*. This increases variation and is one of the reasons why no two individuals (unless they are identical twins) are genetically the same.

chickenpox: see varicella zoster virus.

chimaerism: the mixture of cells* originating from different zygotes* to form a single individual. Chimaeras may be created in research by combining cells from two or more embryos of the same or different strains or species. Combination is usually made by aggregation of cleaving* embryos, or by injection of foreign cells into blastocysts*.

In the UK, creation of human chimaeras is illegal. However any individual who has received a transplant may be considered a chimaera, having genetically unrelated cells coexisting. Chimaeras might result if an oocyte* becomes fertilized by two spermatozoa* and cleaves equally, rather than ejecting the second polar* body, so that a mixture of cell genotypes* is created.

chi-squared test: a very popular test which may, typically, be applied to a contingency* table displaying the frequencies of individuals classified in two or more ways. The test is intended to detect association* between the factors defining the classifications. Since it is an asymptotic, normal theory test, it should not be applied when the expected frequencies in the cells are small (say < 5). An alternate test, Fisher's* exact test, then provides a useful distribution-free * alternative.

The simplest application of the Chi-squared test would perhaps be on a 2 by 2 contingency table, giving perhaps the frequencies (a, b, c, d) of individuals displaying symptoms of two medical conditions.

Thus:

		Condition A	
		No symptoms	Symptoms
Condition B	No symptoms	a	b
	Symptoms	c	d

The test would here determine whether there was evidence of association* between the two medical conditions.

chlamydia trachomatis: this is probably the commonest sexually transmitted bacterium* and causes a wide range of manifestations. In men, it causes non-specific* urethritis (NSU) with symptoms of urethral* discharge and pain on passing urine. It is the commonest cause of epididymo-orchitis* in young men. A considerable proportion, perhaps 50% of men and 90% of women have no symptoms. When present, symptoms in women are mild and may include urinary complaints suggestive of cystitis* and vaginal discharge. Ascent of the infection to the upper genital tract in women is frequent and leads to pelvic* inflammatory disease with the risk of long term damage to the Fallopian* tubes by causing loss of cilia*, scarring, intra-tubal adhesions* or luminal occlusions as well as peri-tubal adhesions*. Chlamydial infection is the commonest cause of tubal infertility and a major cause of extra-uterine* pregnancy.

Transmission of the infection to the baby during delivery can lead to conjunctivitis and, in some infants, pneumonia. Recent studies suggest that chlamydial infection may be associated with pre-term delivery. The diagnosis is made by taking swabs from infected sites and by demonstrating the presence of antibodies* in the blood. Treatment of the active infection with tetracyclines or erythromycin is usually successful. Contact tracing* and treatment of the sexual partner are essential.

chloasma: a patchy yellow or bronze discoloration of the mother's facial skin, often with a mask like distribution, which may occur in pregnancy and usually resolves after delivery. Chloasma can also be caused by the use of oral contraceptives.

chocolate cyst: a form of ovarian endometriosis*; the cysts are lined by functioning endometrium* and filled with a tarry collection of old menstrual blood which resembles thick chocolate sauce. Associated adhesions* are frequent and interfere both with ovulation* and with ovum* pick-up and transport. This form of endometriosis is usually amenable to treatment by open or laparoscopic surgery.

chorio-carcinoma (syn. chorio-epithelioma): a rare malignant uterine* tumour which is derived from trophoblast cells in the chorion*. The majority of these tumours follow a hydatidiform* mole but they can also be preceded by a normal delivery or miscarriage*. Rapidly invasive and early to metastasize (spread), this used to be a virulent cancer leading to early death. It was the first tumour found to respond well to cytotoxic drugs which are now the mainstay of treatment.

chorion: the tougher and outer of the membranes which surround the fetal sac (Fig. 20). It is formed from trophoblast (see trophectoderm) and its outer surface has thousands of small projections, known as chorionic villi, giving it a shaggy appearance. The villi play an essential part in implantation* by invasion of the uterine decidua*, and in transmitting nutrients, waste products and gases between the fetal and the maternal circulations. That part of the chorion which is in contact with the decidua is called the chorion frondosum, retains its villi, and later forms the placenta*. On the aspect of the chorion which projects into the uterine cavity, the villi atrophy and this part of the chorion is known as the chorion laeve.

chorionic gonadotrophin (hCG): the hormone* secreted by the growing chorionic* tissue of the implanting blastocyst* and later by the placenta*: it contains α (alpha) and β (beta) subunits. The α subunit is similar to FSH*, LH* and thyroid stimulating hormone. Presence of the β subunit in blood or urine forms the basis of pregnancy* tests. An injection of human chorionic gonadotrophin (hCG, proprietary names Pregnyl or Profasi) is used in IVF* to mimic the LH* surge*, bring about final maturation of the oocytes* and trigger ovulation*. Oocyte* collection is performed 34–36 hours after the administration of hCG.

chorionic villi: see chorion.

chorionic villus sampling (CVS): a technique employed in the ante-natal diagnosis of chromosomal* disorders, fetal sex and certain other genetic or metabolic defects. Samples of chorionic* villi are aspirated between 10 and 14 weeks of pregnancy, under ultrasound* guidance, either through the cervix* or by abdominal puncture. Compared with amniocentesis*, CVS is performed earlier in pregnancy and results are obtained more quickly, but there is a slightly higher risk of miscarriage*.

chromatid: one of the two strands of chromatin* which together make up one chromosome*. The two chromatids of a chromosome are held together by a centromere* until the cell divides (see anaphase). At this point the two chromatids separate, each going to one of the two daughter cells.

chromatin: the material of which a chromosome* is made. Chromatin consists of DNA* and associated proteins*. Certain histology stains are specific to chromatin. This allows identification of the position, shape and size of chromosomes in a cell.

chromopertubation: a technique employed during diagnostic laparoscopy* to evaluate the tubal status. A coloured solution (usually methylene blue) is injected into the uterine* cavity and the fimbrial* end of the Fallopian* tube is observed through the laparoscope. Escape of dye indicates tubal patency; failure to do so suggests tubal obstruction or spasm.

chromosomes (Fig. 4): the thread-like, darkly staining structures in the cell nucleus* which contain the hereditary material—deoxyribonucleic acid (DNA*)—with associated proteins*. Each chromosome contains an enormously long strand of DNA, coiled and arranged as a double helix, that is like a twisted ladder with uprights and countless rungs.

During most of a cell's life, chromosomes are contracted, existing as

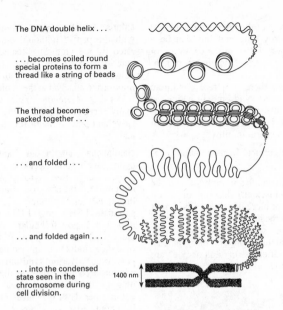

The DNA double helix . . .

. . . becomes coiled round special proteins to form a thread like a string of beads

The thread becomes packed together . . .

. . . and folded . . .

. . . and folded again . . .

. . . into the condensed state seen in the chromosome during cell division.

1400 nm

Fig. **4**. Chromosome. Each chromosome consists of highly folded DNA with associated proteins.

extremely long, thin strands. A cell uses the information contained in its chromosomes to make the proteins and other substances it needs. When a cell is almost ready to divide, its chromosomes coil up into tightly packaged structures which, if stained, are visible under the light microscope. Chromosome duplication involves the replication of DNA and the formation of two identical chromatids* from each chromosome (see mitosis). This is the basis of growth and, in most organs, the repair of dying or damaged cells.

Humans have 46 chromosomes in each of their cells, except for the germ cells (eggs and sperm) which have only 23 as a result of meiosis*. Half of a person's chromosomes come from their mother and half from their father. In chromosome analysis, special techniques are employed to produce a karyotype*, a photographic picture of the chromosomes arranged according to internationally agreed conventions.

chromosomal disorders (*syn.* chromosome mutations): mistakes in chromosome* number or structure. Chromosomal disorders are mainly the result of errors at the time of cell division. They may result in genetic disorders such as Down's* syndrome and Turner's* syndrome. Many major chromosomal disorders are incompatible even with intra-uterine life and result in spontaneous miscarriage*. In women, and to a lesser extent in men, the incidence of chromosome abnormalities in the fetus increases with advancing age* and this is one of the causes of a higher spontaneous miscarriage rate. Some sex chromosome abnormalities result in the live birth of an affected individual (see Klinefelter's and Turner's syndromes). About one in six men with azoospermia* or severely impaired sperm counts have an identifiable chromosome abnormality.

cilia: hair-like projections, found in certain organs on the free surface membrane of epithelial* cells lining a tubular duct. Cilia have the unique property of undulating, i.e. moving forwards and backwards, and thus setting up currents. In humans, they are found lining ducts such as the trachea and bronchi where they prevent the passage of foreign material particles into the lungs. In the female genital tract, ciliated epithelium is found in the Fallopian* tubes and is concerned with ovum* pick-up and transport. Inflammation of the inner lining of the tube (endosalpinx*) may destroy cilia and this can be a contributory factor in the causation of tubal extra-uterine* pregnancy or subfertility.

In men, there is a rare condition, Kartagener's* syndrome, in which the congenital absence of cilia in the bronchial tree is associated with absent or very poor sperm motility.

CIN: see cervical intra-epithelial neoplasia.

cleavage (Fig. 5): in embryology, the mitotic* (asexual) division of a cell into two or more daughter cells. It first occurs in the human embryo* when the unicellular zygote* divides after syngamy*. In the laboratory, this is at least 26 hours after sperm* and oocyte* are mixed *in vitro*.

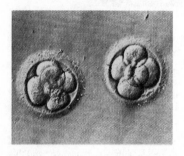

Fig. 5. Cleavage. Cleavage *in vitro* showing two human embryos each with 5 cells.

cleavage stages: the term generally used to mean all stages between 2 cells and compaction* of the embryo. The speed and regularity of cleavage* during this time may be used as an estimate of embryo viability.

climacteric (*syn.* change of life): the phase of life in women, which may extend over several years, when ovarian* activity ceases. The menopause*, i.e. cessation of menstruation, is only one, albeit the most obvious, sign of this process. Other symptoms of oestrogen* deficiency may include hot flushes, night sweats, mood changes, poor concentration and atrophic changes in the vulva* and vagina*. There is no equivalent process in men whose gonadal* activity declines gradually with age; most older men remain potent and fertile.

clitoris: female organ, homologous with the penis* (although not perforated by the urethra), situated in the anterior part of the vulva* (Fig. 27) between the upper folds of the labia* minora and attached to the pubic bones. It consists of erectile tissue, contains many nerve end-organs, is highly sensitive and plays a major role in sexual activity.

clomiphene citrate: an anti-oestrogen*, with some weak oestrogenic properties, used to stimulate ovulation*. It acts on the hypothalamus* and pituitary* gland to stimulate FSH* (and LH*) production and hence follicular* development. Clomiphene is mainly used for ovulation induction in women with polycystic* ovarian syndrome. When administered for 5 days at the beginning of the menstrual cycle (50 to 150 mg per day), it induces ovulation in about 70% of women, but the pregnancy rate is much lower (approximately 30%) and there is a 5% incidence of multiple* pregnancy. Side effects include hot flushes, visual disturbances and abdominal discomfort.

Recent epidemiological data suggest an association between prolonged use of clomiphene and the subsequent development of ovarian* cancer, but such an association has been vigorously denied by other authorities. It is a wise precaution to limit the administration of clomiphene to a maximum of 12 cycles.

clones: a group of individuals that are genetically identical. The HFEA* forbids the formation of human clones, though the production of identical twins from a single zygote* is a form of natural cloning.

co-culture: culture of two or more cell types within the same vessel, sometimes used to support the growth of human embryos* *in vitro*. This usually means the culture of embryos on a layer of other cells (a feeder layer) such as endometrial*, oviductal* or fibroblast cells. The supporting effect of such cells is neither species specific nor restricted to cells from the reproductive tract.

coitus: culmination of sexual activity when the erect penis* is introduced into the vagina* and frictional stimulation between the penis and the vaginal walls occurs, usually leading to ejaculation*. Coitus interruptus is a (poor) method of contraception* where the penis is withdrawn from the vagina before ejaculation to prevent intra-vaginal deposition of semen*.

collagenase: an enzyme* capable of digesting collagen. There are large amounts of collagen in the wall of the ovarian follicle*, and collagenase release is one of the factors which collectively lead to follicular rupture and release of the oocyte* at the time of ovulation*.

colostrum: the clear, sticky fluid secreted by the breasts in late pregnancy and during the first few days after delivery, before the milk flow is established. Colostrum is rich in proteins and fats and contains immunoglobulins* which confer some immunity against infection upon the new-born baby.

colposcope: an instrument incorporating a binocular microscope and light source, used for the examination of body surfaces. It gives a stereoscopic magnification of between 6 and 40 times. The main use for colposcopy is the inspection of the cervix* and vagina* for pre-malignant changes (see carcinoma-in-situ and cervical intra-epithelial neoplasia).

compaction: increasing contact between the blastomeres* of the embryo in late cleavage*, usually at about the 8 to 16 cell stage in humans. The blastomeres adhere closely together to form tight junctions and identification of individual cells becomes impossible.

conception: the process from fusion of the gametes* (see fertilization), through the early development of the conceptus, to implantation* of the blastocyst*.

condom: sheath, made of rubber or other suitable material, which is fitted over the erect penis before coitus. It is often impregnated with a spermicide. This is the oldest and still one of the principal methods of barrier contraception with reasonably good effect when properly used, especially if combined with the use of a spermicidal cream, pessary or foam. Condoms also play a major role in the prevention of spread of sexually* transmitted diseases. A female condom lines the vagina and has the same functions.

Special perforated condoms are available for the collection of semen* from orthodox religious men when masturbation to obtain a sample is forbidden.

condylomata acuminata (genital warts): benign tumours caused by the human* papilloma virus (HPV) and involving any part of the lower genital tract, e.g. introitus*, labia*, vagina* and cervix*, as well as the perineal* and peri-anal region. In men the glans penis*, foreskin, shaft and peri-anal area may be involved.

The condylomata are usually painless, but there may be discharge or irritation. Rapid growth may occur in pregnancy and in the presence of immunosuppression. Treatment is generally unsatisfactory with high recurrence rates irrespective of whether surgery, laser*, diathermy, cryotherapy* or local application of podophyllin compounds are used.

The genital strains of HPV (6 and 11) are sexually transmitted and often found in association with other sexually transmitted diseases*. The association with cervical* or vulval* intra-epithelial neoplasia (pre-invasive carcinoma, CIN* and VIN*) is controversial.

confidence limits: a term describing one measure of the reliability of a statistical estimate of an unknown parameter, such estimate being subject to random variation. Thus the 95% confidence limits define a range within which the analyst is 95% confident that the true, unknown, value of the parameter lies.

confidentiality: the refraining from disclosing personal information, written or spoken, acquired during the performance of professional duties without the permission of the patient or client. All patient-specific medical information has, by tradition, been treated in strict confidence. Confidentiality has assumed increasing significance since the passage of the Human* Fertilisation and Embryology Act (1990) which puts strict limits on the disclosure of certain information by licensed infertility centres. The Act states, with certain exceptions, that information about any identifiable patient who receives treatment services, provides gametes* or is born as a result of treatment services can generally only be disclosed to members and staff of the Authority or to someone else who is covered by a license for the purpose of licensed activities.

Confidentiality generally applies to all medical treatment but also is of particular importance when dealing with conditions such as AIDS*.

congenital malformation (*syn*. birth defect): a fault in a person's anatomy, physiology or biochemistry that is present from their birth. Congenital malformations affect 2–3% of births and may be due to genetic or environmental causes. Examples resulting from genetic causes include Down's* syndrome, cystic fibrosis* and sickle* cell disease. Examples resulting from environmental causes include spina* bifida and fetal* alcohol syndrome* (which can occur if a mother consumes too much alcohol during pregnancy).

consanguinity: blood relationship. Two people are said to be consanguineous if they are related genetically. For instance, half-sibs are consanguineous (since they have one parent in common), whereas a step-child and step-parent are not.

contact tracing (partner notification): this term refers to the confidential* notification of sexual partners of patients with sexually* transmitted diseases that they may be harbouring an infection. The partner is encouraged to seek examination and treatment if appropriate. Contact tracing efforts are crucial in the management of bacterial and viral sexually transmitted diseases, particularly in the prevention of complications in symptom-free individuals.

contingency table: a table of frequencies where individuals are classified according to several discrete* variables. The simplest (2 by 2) contingency table could, typically, provide the frequencies of individuals displaying the presence or absence of two diseases. Larger tables could tabulate the frequencies for numerous discrete random variables at more than two levels.

continuous variable: a variable which can take any value within the permissible range. This contrasts with a discrete* variable which is restricted to specified values (such as integers). Most measurements, such as hormone* concentrations or blood* pressure are continuous variables, whereas the number of oocytes* recovered or the number of embryos* transferred are discrete variables, being confined to integer values.

contraception (*syn*. birth control): the prevention of conception, used to avoid or space pregnancies. The principal methods of contraception are barrier contraception (condom*, vaginal diaphragm, cervical cap), hormonal* contraception (oral contraceptives, depot injections or subcutaneous implants of progestogens*), intra-uterine* contraceptive devices (IUCDs), coitus interruptus (see coitus) and the 'safe period'. The last two, although used most commonly and world wide, are the least effective. Sterilization* has in the last decade become one of the most widely used methods of contraception and is generally achieved in women by various operations on the Fallopian* tubes and in men by vasectomy*.

Emergency contraception, also known as post-coital contraception or the 'morning-after' pill (incorrectly since it is effective for up to 72 hours after intercourse) can be used to prevent conception after unprotected intercourse (e.g. contraception failure, rape). This is achieved by the use of oral contraceptive hormones, up to 72 hours after intercourse, or insertion of an IUCD within five days of intercourse.

cord: see umbilical cord.

cornu: (lit. horn. Fig. 26) the location in the uterus* where the interstitial portion of the Fallopian* tube* enters the endometrial* cavity and which corresponds to the uterine horn in lower mammals. Infections, endometriosis* or polyps* can cause partial or complete cornual occlusion, thus interfering with transport of spermatozoa* or zygotes* and causing infertility or cornual (extra-uterine) pregnancy. (See also utero–tubal junction.)

corona radiata (Fig. 17): the innermost cumulus*-granulosa cells surrounding the oocyte* and its zona* pellucida. The corona cells are initially closely apposed to the zona pellucida and have cytoplasmic* extensions crossing the zona and in direct contact with the membrane of the immature oocyte. The action of cumulus and corona cells prevents premature maturation and supports the oocyte's nutrition. As the oocyte matures, the cellular connections are withdrawn and the corona cells produce mucus, pushing them apart and away from the oocyte and giving the appearance of radiating away (hence corona radiata). The corona cells remain attached to the zona pellucida during ovulation*, but are lost within a day or two.

corpus albicans (Fig. 11): the whitish scarred area on the surface of the ovary* which remains following the disintegration of the corpus* luteum.

corpus cavernosum: one of the two columns of sponge-like erectile tissue found in the clitoris and penis. These columns are surrounded by the ischiocavernosus muscles which, by contracting, trap blood and cause stiffening and erection of the organ.

corpus luteum (Fig. 11): a yellow structure formed in the ovary* after rupture of the Graafian follicle* and expulsion of the oocyte*. It results from changes in the granulosa* and theca* interna cells which produce a yellow pigment called lutein. The fully formed corpus luteum is approximately 2 cm in diameter and secretes progesterone*. It grows and continues to be active during the first 3–4 months of pregnancy. If there has been no conception*, the cells degenerate, progesterone production ceases, menstruation ensues and eventually all that remains is a small white scarred area on the surface of the ovary, known as the corpus albicans*.

correlation: a term widely used to describe the interdependence of two or more variables. Correlation tends to be used more for continuous* variables, whereas association * is often used for discrete* variables.

cortical granules: small membrane-bound particles positioned near the surface of the mature oocyte* and containing trypsin-like enzymes*. At fertilization, the granules fuse with the ovarian membrane, release their contents and so render the zona* pellucida impermeable to further sperm* penetration. This is the so-called 'zona reaction' which ensures that only one spermatozoon may fertilize the oocyte.

cortisone: a hormone* produced by the adrenal* cortex. It is available therapeutically as cortisone acetate and its synthetic analogues include prednisone. It is used for the suppression of reaction to stress and, by virtue of its anti-inflammatory effect, in diseases such as rheumatoid arthritis and ulcerative colitis. Cortisone antagonizes insulin and raises glucose concentrations; in large doses it causes sodium retention and potassium depletion.

Corticosteroids can be used to treat men with immunological* infertility due to antisperm* antibodies, but they have significant side effects such as gastro-intestinal bleeding, precipitation of diabetes*, weight gain and osteoporosis*.

cotyledon: one of approximately 20 lobes, divided by deep fissures, on the uterine surface of the placenta*. Each cotyledon contains major branches of the umbilical* cord vessels for the transport of gases, nutrients and waste products, to and from the fetus.

counselling: a process which seeks to help persons in distress and which can be applied to any branch of medicine where patients suffer trauma and distress and need help in resolving difficulties which interfere with decision making. Counselling is a key element in the provision of infertility services and is distinct from discussions with a doctor related to the giving of information, treatment or consent. It is an approach which looks behind the obvious, tries to understand what goes on in people's minds, and how external factors can stand in the way of decision making and change. It tries to isolate factors and bring them in the open so that people can better understand their emotions, have the strength to tackle their difficulties and be comfortable with their decisions. It does not seek to provide answers but is there to help individuals find their own solutions and respect their decisions.

Fertility clinics in the UK must be licensed by the HFEA* if they provide treatment which involves the use of donor gametes* or IVF*. Part of the requirement for a license is that counselling is provided by trained and experienced counsellors. The HFEA identifies three major areas of counselling in assisted reproductive medicine:
• Implication counselling: this aims to enable people to understand the implications of proposed courses of treatment for themselves, their families and for any children which may be born as a result of such treatment. This is particularly important where IVF*, egg* donation, donor* insemination, freezing* and storing of gametes* and embryos* and micro-injection* are proposed.
• Support counselling: this recognises the emotional needs and stresses which childlessness and fertility treatment impose, particularly at times of failure.
• Therapeutic counselling: this seeks to help people cope with the consequences of treatment and help them to resolve any problems which may arise, drawing upon their own strength and resources. It includes helping people understand their expectations, to work within their resources (financial, emotional, spiritual, time etc.) and to adjust to their situation—including the prospect of adjusting to childlessness where fertility treatment has failed. (See also genetic counselling.)

crossmatch: term for the laboratory procedure when donated blood is selected as being compatible for a particular patient requiring transfusion. (See blood groups.)

cryopreservation: the storage of gametes* or embryos* by freezing at low temperature. Frozen samples are usually stored in straws, vials or ampoules in liquid nitrogen at −196°C in order to prevent destruction by bacterial action or biochemical change. In the UK a license fom the HFEA* is required for units undertaking cryopreservation and storage of human spermatozoa, embryos or oocytes.

Spermatozoa: semen* samples are usually prepared and diluted with a buffered cryoprotectant, such as egg yolk, and are then loaded into vials or straws and placed directly into liquid nitrogen vapour (approximately −80°C) to freeze, before plunging into liquid nitrogen. In general, sperm freezing leads to a 50% reduction in fertility potential, but in a normal sample sufficient spermatozoa will remain viable on thawing for most types of insemination. Sperm can be frozen for various reasons, including quarantine before donor* insemination, possible sterility from radiotherapy or chemotherapy in cancer treatment, before vasectomy* as insurance against marital breakdown and, in assisted conception, to provide a readily available reservoir of the husband's sperm at the time of oocyte* collection. Freezing can also be used in cases of obstructive* or secretory azoospermia* when surgical sperm collection can be conveniently organized in advance of an ICSI* cycle.

Embryos: pre-implantation embryos may be cryopreserved successfully as zygotes*, cleavage* stages or blastocysts*. They are usually frozen slowly at a controlled rate in the presence of a cryoprotectant e.g. 1,2-propanediol (PrOH), di-methyl sulphoxide (DMSO) or glycerol, and/or a dehydrating agent such as sucrose. Some embryos are damaged during freeze–thaw because of intracellular ice formation, gas bubble formation or physical disruption by ice chards. Cleavage stage embryos can lose some cells (usually less than half the total number) through damage and still retain their potential for development. Embryos damaged at the blastocyst stage rarely implant. Embryos are usually cryopreserved when a woman has more available than are required for transfer to the uterus on one occasion, or from women at risk of developing ovarian* hyperstimulation syndrome (OHSS) in whom embryo transfer is contra-indicated. Additional reasons given under the entry for 'spermatozoa' above, may also apply. In the UK, initially embryos could legally be kept in storage for transfer up to 5 years. This was extended in 1996 to 10 years, providing consent for the extension is obtained from both partners.

Oocytes: these can be frozen and thawed in the same way as embryos; however, they usually become resistant to fertilization*. The stage of the oocyte may be important as the cytoskeleton can be very sensitive to cooling, and disruption of the spindle on which the chromatids* are arranged in mature oocytes might be detrimental to subsequent development. This method is therefore rarely used, although research in this area is continuing. The ability to cryopreserve oocytes and retain their fertility would greatly improve the clinical options for girls and women facing sterilizing treatment (oophorectomy*, irradiation, chemotherapy), as well as improving the management of egg* donation.

cryoprotectant: substance added to cells which reduces damage during freezing and thawing (see cryopreservation). Examples include 1,2-propanediol, dimethyl sulphoxide, glycerol, egg yolk.

cryosurgery: the use of cold by freezing or liquid nitrogen to destroy tissue. It can be used in the treatment of CIN* and ectropion* of the cervix* and of genital warts (see condyloma).

crypto-azoospermia: apparent azoospermia* on routine semen* analysis but a very small number of spermatozoa are found after high speed centrifugation of the semen. Cryptoazoospermic samples may be used successfully for intra-cytoplasmic* sperm injection to produce embryos *in vitro* in the treatment of severe male factor infertility.

cryptomenorrhoea (*lit.* hidden menstruation): this occurs when endometrial * shedding takes place but the menstrual* loss cannot escape due to blockage of parts of the lower genital tract. Whilst the occlusion may be at the cervix* or in the upper vagina*, by far the commonest site is an imperforate hymen*. The patient presents with a history of primary amenorrhoea* but menstrual symptoms are usually present and on examination a pelvic and/or lower abdominal mass is found, consisting of the distended vagina, uterus and tubes, filled with old blood. Treatment is by incision of the thickened hymen

cryptorchidism: see undescended testes.

culture medium: a solution in which cells* can be grown *in vitro*. Culture media must be the same osmolarity (strength) as body fluids, and contain various substances necessary for the cells' survival, including serum, protein or a protein substitute such as a polymer. Culture media used successfully for oocytes*, spermatozoa* and embryos* range from very simple balanced salt solutions (e.g. Earle's medium, acid* Tyrode solution) to complex media (e.g.Ham's, Bigger's) which may contain amino-acids, antioxidants, hormones*, vitamins and other biologically active compounds.

cumulative conception rate (CCR): conception* rates after certain events, such as discontinuation of oral contraceptives or IUCDs*, tubal surgery or IVF*, were traditionally calculated by dividing the number of patients who have conceived by the total number of patients studied or treated. This is an unsatisfactory measure of outcome as it underestimates the number of conceptions by excluding patients lost to follow-up and those who entered a trial shortly before its closure.

Cumulative conception rates, calculated on an actuarial basis by means of life time table analysis, aim to provide an estimate of the progressive success of an ongoing treatment. For the figure to be truly reliable, a cohort of patients needs to be studied throughout the treatment period. Radical assumptions have to be made to overcome the problem of patients 'dropping-out'. Typical is the assumption that the conception rate for the drop-outs is no different from that of the patients who remain in the study.Whilst many clinicians now consider the CCRs to be the best index of outcome in infertility treatments, some statisticians regard them as being rather optimistic estimates.

cumulus oophorus: cluster of specialized granulosa* cells around the oocyte* in antral follicles*. During follicle growth, the cumulus cells protect and nourish the oocyte, and the inner corona* cells communicate directly with it via gap junctions. The cumulus cells also help to prevent premature maturation of the oocyte. During the time between the LH* surge and ovulation*, the cumulus in ripe follicles expands and becomes mucified. The cumulus mass assists in the ovum* pick-up process by the Fallopian tube and its expansion is believed to assist sperm capacitation* and access to the oocyte. The degree of cumulus expansion may be used in embryology to estimate oocyte maturity, although wide discrepancies between oocyte maturity and cumulus maturity may be present after hormonal stimulation of follicle growth.

curettage: removal of part of the endometrial* lining of the uterus by means of a hollow spoon-shaped instrument (curette). Dilatation of the cervix* is required to admit all but the smallest curette. This operation is a diagnostic procedure to study hormonal or other changes (inflammatory, neoplastic) in the endometrial cells, or a therapeutic procedure for the removal of retained* products of conception or uterine polyps*.

Cushing's syndrome: this condition results from an excess secretion of adrenal* cortical hormones (mainly cortisol), caused either by a basophil adenoma* of the anterior lobe of the pituitary* gland or by hyperplasia* or tumours of the adrenal cortex. Clinical signs in both sexes include obesity (limited to the trunk), reddening of the face and neck, stretch marks in the skin, hirsutism* and hypertension. Diabetes*, osteoporosis* and hyperprolactinaemia* frequently develop. In women, there is amenorrhoea*.

cyesis: syn. pregnancy*.

cyproterone acetate: a drug which blocks the action of androgens* and is used for the treatment of hirsutism* or acne in women. It is also used in men in the treatment of prostate* cancer or abnormally high libido*.

cyst: a cavity with fluid or semi-solid contents. This is a very common condition which can affect virtually any organ. *Retention cysts* are due to blockage of a duct with accumulation of fluid, e.g. Bartholin's cyst. *Congenital cysts* contain embryonic material, e.g. Gärtner's duct cyst or ovarian dermoid*. *Inclusion cysts* are formed from small fragments of skin or mucous membrane buried beneath the surface, following injury (e.g. vaginal laceration during labour) or surgery. Many cysts are due to *benign neoplastic* changes. These are particularly common in glandular organs such as breast or ovary. *Chocolate* cysts of the ovary* are not neoplastic, but the result of bleeding from functioning endometrial implants (endometriosis*) on the surface of the ovary, and are associated with infertility. Ovarian follicular* and corpus* luteum cysts are associated with hormonal upsets.

Many cysts are asymptomatic. Others may present as a 'lump' or with an acute complication such as torsion or a haemorrhage into the cyst: the latter is particularly common in a corpus luteum cyst and can cause symptoms and signs similar to an extrauterine* pregnancy. Most cysts can be visualized by ultrasound*.

In men, small cysts of the epididymis* may contain spermatozoa* and are called spermatoceles*, whilst cysts of the spermatic* cord, 'hydroceles*, do not contain spermatozoa.

cystic fibrosis: a hereditary condition caused by a recessive* allele* so that only people who have two abnormal alleles in each of their nuclei* are affected by the condition. On average one in every 24 white Europeans carries the allele which means that one in 2000 children born to white European parents has cystic fibrosis. A person with cystic fibrosis produces abnormally thick mucus, particularly in the lungs, pancreas and digestive tract. Vigorous physiotherapy is needed daily to help prevent pulmonary infections and patients have to take pancreatic enzymes with every meal to aid digestion. In the 1950s babies born with cystic fibrosis usually died within a year or two of birth. By the 1970s people born with cystic fibrosis had a life expectancy of around 20–30 years. The advent of gene* therapy, heart and lung transplants and advances in conventional medicine mean that the prospects for people with cystic fibrosis leading a long and fairly healthy life are improving rapidly.

cystitis: inflammation of the urinary bladder. This is very common in women due to the short length of the urethra* and may be associated with incomplete emptying of the bladder, ascending infection provoked by sexual activity or catheterization, or by downward tracking from a kidney infection (pyelonephritis). The condition may be acute or chronic, and presents with symptoms of pain on urination, frequency and a constant desire to pass urine. Blood in the urine may be due to cystitis. A specimen of urine is usually obtained for laboratory examination. The commonest cause is an *E. coli* bacterial infection which usually responds well to treatment with antibiotics.

In men, cystitis is rare, but may be associated with prostatic* enlargement, kidney stones and other conditions which require full investigation.

cytokines: a large group of molecules secreted by many cells*, but particularly T lymphocytes and macrophages. They include interferons and interleukins and have diverse biological effects. In general terms they can be thought of as hormones* that act at short range (though some do have systemic effects). Their primary role appears to be in the regulation of the immune* response, though other roles in the regulation of growth and differentiation and the interaction between the secretory endometrium* and early embryo* during implantation* have been identified.

cytomegalovirus: a herpes* virus* which may cause severe disease in babies. Infection with cytomegalovirus is common; by childbearing age between 40% and 80% of the population have been exposed to the virus. An active cytomegalovirus infection can occur as a primary infection at the time of first exposure or as reactivation in which latent (dormant) virus begins to replicate once more. The infant suffers serious consequences (including mental retardation and liver problems) in around 5% of primary infections occurring in pregnant women, but these rarely occur as a result of reactivation

cytoplasm: the contents of a cell* between the outer membrane and the nuclear membrane. The cytoplasm of the oocyte* is called ooplasm.

cytotrophoblast (*syn.* Langhans layer): the inner layer of cells lining the early chorionic* villi (the outer layer is called the syncytio-trophoblast*). The cytotrophoblast is entirely fetal in origin and forms a membrane across which the exchange of blood gases, nutrients and waste products between mother and fetus takes place; it disappears after the fifth month of pregnancy.

D

Danazol: a synthetic, orally active testosterone* analogue which inhibits pituitary gonadotrophins* and so suppresses oestrogen* and progesterone* secretion. It is used in the treatment of endometriosis* to produce a 'pseudomenopause', i.e. amenorrhoea* and suppression of ovulation*. This relieves pain and dyspareunia*. Side effects include reversible increase in weight, hirsutism* and acne. Voice changes may be permanent. Earlier optimism about the success of treating endometriosis-related infertility with Danazol is being questioned. It is of little help in the management of patients with structural changes (adhesions) resulting from the more severe grades of endometriosis, or with chocolate* cysts.

decidua (Fig. 20): the altered uterine lining (endometrium*) in pregnancy, when it becomes thicker, more vascular and the glands become more prominent with greater secretory activity, so that implantation* can occur. The decidua sustains the blastocyst* during implantation and its early development by producing nutrition and adhesives.

The decidua basalis is that area of uterine wall where the developing embryo implants and the placenta* will develop. The decidua capsularis covers the developing blastocyst, isolating it from the uterine cavity; the rest of the lining of the uterus is known as decidua parietalis or vera.

decidual cast: in an extra-uterine* pregnancy the endometrium* undergoes decidual* changes under the influence of early pregnancy hormones, but contains no villi* as there has been no intra-uterine implantation. When the ectopic pregnancy fails, or is removed surgically, the hormonal changes regress and the decidualized endometrium is expelled, often in a single piece as a complete 'cast' of the uterine cavity.

decondensation: the conversion of the spermatozoon* into the male pronucleus*. The sperm nucleus* is extremely compact and the chromatids* are held together very tightly by protamines. Once the sperm enters the ooplasm* at fertilization*, its nucleus must decondense in an orderly fashion from its highly compacted state so that the nuclear material can become accessible for pronucleus formation and syngamy*.

delayed fertilization: fertilization which occurs later than the usual approximately 18 hour period between insemination and pronucleus* formation in human oocytes* *in vitro*. Delayed fertilization results in embryos less competent to develop further than those fertilized promptly.

Delayed fertilization is normal in some species such as certain bats where the females store semen* in the uterus* following mating in autumn, but do not relax the utero–tubal* junction to allow passage of spermatozoa into the Fallopian* tube until the following spring.

delayed implantation: implantation* of the embryo* after a period of arrested development known as diapause. This phenomenon does not occur in humans but can ocur in badgers, some deer and some rodents. Blastocysts* rest in the uterus* without implanting and may remain so for days or weeks before hormonal changes in the mother stimulate them to implant.

deletion: the loss of DNA* in chromosomes*. Deletions may be of only a few bases (see DNA) or of many genes*. Deletions result from mistakes at cell division. By and large, the more genes are affected the more serious the consequences. Long deletions are rarely compatible with life.

density gradient: a method of preparing spermatozoa* for assisted* reproduction techniques by centrifuging seminal* fluid through layers of fine particles in order to filter out debris, dead spermatozoa and abnormal cells. The gradients are layers of particles of colloidal silica coated by polyvinylpyrrolidone (PVP), prepared in a centrifuge tube. Semen is placed above the gradient which is then centrifuged for 20 minutes. The small sperm pellet formed at the bottom of the tube is then aspirated and used for insemination. (See also sperm preparation.)

depot provera: see medroxyprogesterone.

dermoid cyst: a benign ovarian tumour containing skin elements including hair follicles, sebaceous glands and teeth. Other structures such as bone, cartilage or glandular tissue may be present. The cyst is filled with thick, yellow, greasy sebaceous fluid. Dermoids are common and constitute 10 to 15% of all ovarian tumours. They are often bilateral. They are usually asymptomatic and patients present with gradually increasing abdominal enlargement or an acute complication such as torsion. They are often diagnosed at a routine examination or ultrasound* scan in pregnancy or in infertility investigations. Treatment is surgical, with excision of the cyst whilst aiming to preserve some normal functioning ovarian tissue (ovarian cystectomy).

determination: the point at which the developmental fate of a particular cell* is decided. Cells may be determined to follow a particular type of development according to their location and the developmental fates of their neighbouring cells.

diabetes mellitus: a common disorder of carbohydrate metabolism associated with lack of, or resistance to, the pancreatic hormone*, insulin. High blood sugar concentrations and disturbed acid/base balance result and may cause diabetic coma. Insulin-dependent (type I) diabetes usually presents in childhood, adolescence or below the age of 40.

Diabetes may develop for the first time in pregnancy (gestational diabetes) and can cause problems in the management of the pregnant woman and her fetus. It is doubtful whether women with well controlled diabetes have an increased incidence of infertility or miscarriage.

Male diabetics may have erectile impotence* or retrograde* ejaculation.

diakinesis: one of the stages at the beginning of meiosis*.

didelphys uterus (Fig. 16): the presence of two uteri*, two cervices and a double vagina, resulting from failure of fusion of the lower parts of the Müllerian* ducts. This condition can be visualized by ultrasound*, hysterosalpingography* or hysteroscopy*. It is usually asymptomatic and diagnosed on gynaecological examination or in pregnancy. It is not a cause of infertility but may cause complications in pregnancy or labour, such as miscarriage*, malpresentation, post-partum haemorrhage or retained placenta.

diethyl stilboestrol (DES): the first orally active substance with oestrogenic* effect, synthesized by Charles Dodds in 1938. It was widely used initially in the treatment of amenorrhoea*, menopausal* symptoms and for suppression of lactation* because it was cheap, easy to produce, could be taken by mouth and was more potent than natural oestrogens. Subsequently it was used, mainly in the USA, in the mistaken idea that it might prevent certain pregnancy complications. However, intra-uterine exposure of the fetus to DES administered to the mother in pregnancy led to abnormal cellular changes in the vagina* and cervix*, some cases of vaginal adenocarcinoma, as well as structural malformations of the genital tract in both female and male fetuses.

This was the first time it was realized that a drug administered to a woman in pregnancy could cause permanent damage and even malignant changes in the fetus.

differentiation: the point occurring after determination* at which cells become different from each other, as they initiate development into distinct cell types. In the embryo the initial differentiation is probably into outside (polar) and inside (apolar) cells which will later form the trophectoderm* and inner* cell mass respectively. As cells differentiate, totipotency, present during cleavage*, is lost.

dilatation of the cervix: this occurs naturally in labour and in spontaneous miscarriages* when uterine contractions, associated with sustained shortening of the muscle fibres (retraction), cause first shortening of the cervical canal ('taking up' or 'effacement') and then progressive enlargement of its opening, to allow the fetus to pass from uterus to vagina. Dilatation is performed surgically with graduated dilators prior to curettage*. For this, regional or general anaesthesia is usually employed.

diploid cell: a cell with two sets of chromosomes*, one from the mother and one from the father. In humans, diploid cells contain 46 chromosomes. All the cells in a human are diploid with the exception of the gametes* (spermatozoa* and oocytes*) which have only 23 chromosomes, certain cells which lack a nucleus (such as red blood cells) and a few cells (including some found in the liver) which have three or more sets of chromosomes.

direct intra-peritoneal injection (DIPI): see intra-peritoneal insemination.

discrete variable: a variable where the values are restricted to a specified set within the admissible range. Typically these could be integers (1, 2, etc.). The analysis of discrete data generally requires different statistical methods from those used for continuous* variables, especially if the range of values is small.

dizygotic twins (binovular twins): non-identical twins resulting from the fertilization* of two oocytes*. This may occur spontaneously or after ovarian* stimulation and assisted conception. The resulting children resemble each other no more than other siblings and may be of different sex.

DNA (deoxyribonucleic acid, Fig. 6): the basic biological molecule of heredity and of the control of many cellular functions. It is located largely in chromosomes* and also in mitochondria*, centrioles and other organelles in the cytoplasm*.

Human cells contain 46 functioning DNA molecules—one for each chromosome. DNA has a repetitive structure, consisting of a constant 'backbone', arranged as a double helix,

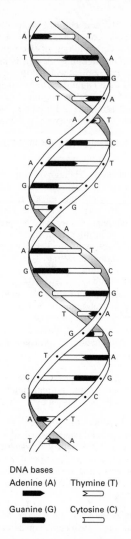

DNA bases

Adenine (A) Thymine (T)

Guanine (G) Cytosine (C)

Fig. 6. DNA. The chemical structure of DNA, showing the double helix.

from which project chemicals known as bases. There are four different bases found in DNA, abbreviated A, C, G and T. It is the order of these bases that determines the chemical structures of all the materials made in the cell.

DNA can be thought of as an alphabet with just four letters. These four letters make up a total of 64 three-letter 'words'. These 64 words (AAA, AAC, AAG and AAT to give just four of them) are themselves gathered together to make 'sentences', called genes*. A typical gene might have a hundred or so words, i.e. around three hundred bases. Each gene is responsible for the manufacture by the cell of a different protein*.

Humans probably have somewhere between 50 000 and 100 000 functioning genes. Our genes help to make us who we are. With the exception of identical twins, no two people have exactly the same order of bases in their DNA. It is the fact that identical twins do have precisely the same order of bases in their DNA that makes a pair of identical twins so similar to each other.

dominance: in a normal diploid* cell, the alleles* that make up a gene* are found in pairs, one allele being maternal in origin, the other paternal. An allele is said to be dominant when it has its effect irrespective of whether it is inherited from only one parent or from both. For example, the allele responsible for Huntington's* chorea is dominant. (See also recessive.)

donor insemination (DI): artificial insemination using donated semen*: previously known as AID, this is now referred to as DI, in order to avoid confusion with AIDS*. This is a very successful treatment for male infertility.

Cryopreserved* semen is stored in sperm banks, licensed by the HFEA*. The donors recruited are usually medical students or other university undergraduates who receive no payment other than reimbursement of expenses. In the UK, donors are registered with the HFEA who limit to ten the number of children a donor may father and who also record non-identifying characteristics such as occupation; education; race; skin, eye and hair colour; height; build; medical history and blood group. Only such non-identifying information can be provided at a later date by the HFEA to children conceived from donor sperm. It also enables the tracing of donors in the event of clinical need and so that a child on reaching the age of 18 (or earlier if they marry) can ask the Authority if there is a danger of their marrying a relative.

All donors undergo tests for infection (see HIV), chromosome* studies and a test to eliminate cystic* fibrosis carrier status. Spermatozoa* may be donated for the treatment of couples with severe male factor infertility (including some cancer patients treated with radiotherapy or chemotherapy), and in certain cases of hereditary disease. Insemination can be by artificial* insemination, IVF* or GIFT*. Counselling* should be available to help couples explore and be comfortable with the implications of DI. Couples will want to explore the selection of donors, screening, matching, legal consequences, definitions of 'father' and whether they will tell the child about its genetic origins. Donors have no responsibility or liability towards any future children and are not to be considered as the father. As surgical* sperm retrieval and micro-injection* techniques are being improved, the need for DI is diminishing.

dopamine: a neuro-hormone* produced in the part of the brain known as the hypothalamus*; together with GnRH* it regulates the pituitary* secretion of FSH*, LH* and prolactin*. Dopamine functions as a prolactin* inhibitory factor and is raised in women with hyperprolactinaemia*. This results in suppression of hypothalamic* and pituitary* function, leading to amenorrhoea* and anovulation*. Hyperprolactinaemia is treated with dopamine agonists (see bromocriptine*).

Doppler: 19th century astronomer who studied light emission from stars and found changes in colour due to changes in the relative movement of the light source and observer. Similar changes in the frequency of sound waves bounced back from rapidly moving bodily targets, such as blood cells, are used in ultrasonography*, for example in the study of uterine, placental, umbilical or testicular blood flow and in studies of the fetal circulation, to assess the status of the fetus. Doppler is also used in the clinical diagnosis of varicoceles*.

Douglas, pouch of: see pouch of Douglas.

Down's syndrome: (previously known as Mongolism): a congenital abnormality due to a chromosomal* disorder: the majority of cases are due to trisomy*

21 and are associated with increasing maternal age*, with a frequency of about 1:2000 at the age of 20, 1:100 at 40 and 1:40 at 45. However, because far more young women have babies, Down's syndrome is commoner in babies born to younger mothers. Increasing paternal age is also relevant but much less so. A small number of cases (about 4%) are associated with a translocation* usually involving chromosomes 21 and 14: this may arise *de novo* or be associated with a balanced translocation (see Robertsonian translocation) in either parent in which case there is a 1:3 risk of recurrence in further children.

Clinically, a Down's syndrome child has a broad flat face, with obliquely placed eyes, enlarged epicanthic folds, small nose and thick lips. There is considerable mental disability, though the severity varies. There is a high incidence of congenital heart disease or duodenal atresia.

Maternal age above 35/36 years or a history of previous occurrence were the major indications for amniocentesis* and chorionic* villus sampling when these were first introduced. More recently screening by measuring serum alpha-feto* protein and hCG* (double test) or including oestriol* (triple test) has been introduced. Ultrasound* to measure the thickness of the fluid at the back of the fetal neck ('nuchal translucency') is also used as a screening technique. Both the serum and the ultrasound screening tests have a high incidence of false positives which can lead to an increase in the number of amniocenteses performed and also to greater parental anxiety.

drug effects on fertility: these are either intentional (e.g. fertility drugs to promote pregnancy, contraceptive preparations to prevent pregnancy, cyproterone* acetate to reduce male libido), or are side effects which generally inhibit, rather than promote, fertility.

Both oogenesis* and spermatogenesis* can be impaired by chemotherapy and a wide variety of other commonly prescribed medications. In addition in men, impotence* may be caused by certain diuretics, beta-blockers, hypotensives, antidepressants, alcohol abuse, marihuana and many other preparations. Ejaculation* failure or retrograde* ejaculation can also be caused by a variety of drugs, including certain hypotensives and antidepressants.

drugs, relating to pregnancy: most drugs cross the placental* barrier and many pass into the milk: however dilution in the mother's body makes the latter route of transmission less significant. In pregnancy, the exact time of fetal exposure to drugs administered to the mother may determine the type and severity of any fetal abnormalities. DES (diethyl* stilboestrol) was the first transplacental carcinogen discovered: fortunately only about 1 in 1000 exposed fetuses were affected. Thalidomide* was the first drug given to mothers that was found to be teratogenic*. When given between days 21 and 36 after conception, there was an almost 100% likelihood of major fetal malformations. Other drugs which can have significant effects on the fetus include cytotoxic drugs, anticonvulsants, certain anticoagulants, some hormones and steroids*, alcohol* and by-products of smoking*. Narcotics and drugs of addiction (heroin, cocaine) also have harmful effects on the fetus and newborn. However, only about 1% of congenital abnormalities are attributable to teratogenic drugs ingested in pregnancy.

Duchenne muscular dystrophy: one of a group of muscular disorders which is hereditary and sex-linked*, and so is found in boys and almost never in girls. There is progressive weakness and atrophy of the muscles of the trunk and limbs, leading to severe disability and, usually, death in adolescence. About two-thirds of cases are the result of inheriting the faulty allele* from the mother; the other third are the result of new mutations*.

Until the mid-1990s, avoidance was only by pre-natal sex diagnosis with termination of all pregnancies with a male fetus. Pre-implantation* diagnosis by genetic testing of embryonic biopsies is now feasible in cases selected because of the previous occurrence of an affected child. This avoids the need for (often late) pregnancy termination. Another advantage over pre-natal sex diagnosis is that half the male fetuses aborted as a result of pre-natal diagnosis are healthy.

Dysmenorrhoea: painful menstruation. Primary (*syn*. spasmodic) dysmenorrhoea starts at or soon after the menarche*, consists of colicky pain on day 1 of the flow, and may be accompanied by nausea, vomiting, diarrhoea, sweating and faintness. Secondary (*syn*. congestive) dysmenorrhoea is seen later in life in women not necessarily previously affected, and usually exhibits pain starting before the onset of the flow and possibly relieved by it. This form of dysmenorrhoea is usually associated with pelvic* inflammatory disease, endometriosis* or reaction of the uterus to fibroid* polyps or IUCDs*.

dyspareunia: pain during intercourse. In women, superficial dyspareunia may be due to inflammation of the vulva* or vagina*, deficient lubrication, vaginismus* or scarring following lacerations sustained at a previous delivery. Deep dyspareunia is associated with pelvic* inflammatory disease, endometriosis* or occasionally uterine retroversion*.

In men pain during intercourse may be due to phimosis* (tight foreskin) or a tight frenulum (the skin fold joining the undersurface of the glans penis* to the foreskin). Pain on ejaculation* can be caused by a urethral stricture, epididymitis*, chronic prostatitis* or a sperm granuloma which may follow surgery on the vas* deferens.

Dyspareunia is a very important symptom in infertility investigations: apart from pointing to a diagnosis of the cause of the infertility, it may also reduce the frequency of intercourse or the depth of penetration, causing failure of semen* deposition near the cervix*.

E

Earle's medium: see culture medium.

early pregnancy loss: miscarriage* in the first trimester* of pregnancy (i.e. up to the 13th week). Very early pregnancy loss due to implantation* failure is frequently not recognized. There may be no, or only slight, menstrual delay, with perhaps a heavier loss than usual.This may be associated with only a transitory rise in hCG* and no fetus is seen on ultrasound* scanning. Such 'biochemical* pregnancies' or 'preclinical miscarriages' are frequently detected after IVF* and occur in 15 to 20% of patients after embryo* transfer.

Early pregnancy loss, involving an established pregnancy, occurs in at least 15% of all pregnancies. A threatened miscarriage may present as painless bleeding in early pregnancy. This may resolve with the pregnancy continuing normally. If pain and heavy bleeding ensue, the miscarriage beomes inevitable. Some women may go on to miscarry completely at home, in which case bleeding and pain will stop once the uterus* is empty. Many however will continue having pain, bleeding and the intermittent passage of placental* tissue and will require hospital admission for pain relief and evacuation of retained* products of conception (ERPC) under general anaesthesia. This condition is known as incomplete miscarriage. Fetal death may be a chance finding on a routine ultrasound scan. This is known as a missed abortion. The woman may have noticed disappearance of early pregnancy symptoms such as nausea and breast tenderness. Missed abortion may be managed conservatively, i.e. by waiting for the uterus to empty naturally, but this can take days or even weeks, and an ERPC may be advised as an alternative.

The incidence of early pregnancy loss is directly related to maternal age*: it increases after 35 and steeply after 40 years. The incidence is also increased in women who have had one or more previous miscarriages (see recurrent miscarriage). The majority of sporadic early pregnancy losses are associated with fetal chromosomal* abnormalities which prevent development of a normal fetus. Multiple* conceptions, maternal infections, abnormalities of the maternal genital tract, hormonal and immunological* factors are rarer causes.

Women who suffer early pregnancy loss require consideration and sympathy. Many feel guilty and blame themselves or external events. Significant anniversaries such as the date the baby would have been due, had the pregnancy continued, may be emotionally traumatic and should be explained to the couple. Most doctors would advise waiting until normal menstruation restarts before trying to conceive again. (See also miscarriage, abortion, blighted ovum.)

eclampsia: convulsions, similar to fits seen in epilepsy, occurring in pregnancy, labour or after delivery, and usually preceded by pre-eclampsia*. Coma usually follows the fits and without treatment the fits can re-occur. Magnesium sulphate is now regarded as the treatment of choice. This is a very dangerous condition for mother and fetus with a high maternal and perinatal mortality* rate. Most cases can be prevented by good antenatal and intra-partum care and early treatment of pre-eclampsia.

ectopic pregnancy: see extra-uterine pregnancy.

ectropion: pouting of the lips of the cervix* so that the external* cervical os is enlarged, irregular and patulous; this is the result of lacerations (usually bilateral) of the cervix in labour or during forcible dilatation*. Ectropion is usually asymptomatic, but may be associated with chronic cervicitis and even an ascending endometritis* in which case surgical repair is indicated.

egg: see oocyte, ovum.

egg donation (oocyte or ovum donation): eggs from one woman may be given to another woman to help her achieve a pregnancy. Eggs may also be donated for research. Initially egg donation was only used for women who produced no eggs because of congenital abnormalities (e.g. Turner's* syndrome) or premature* ovarian failure. Donation is now also employed in certain cases of hereditary disease, repeated early* pregnancy loss, infertility due to surgical or chemotherapeutic removal of the ovaries, and even advanced maternal age*.

Eggs are collected from the donor (as for IVF*), usually after ovarian* stimulation, and are fertilized with the recipient's partner's spermatozoa *in vitro*. The resultant embryo is transferred to the recipient's uterus. The donor may be related to the recipient, though this is discouraged in the UK. Other sources of oocytes are volunteers, patients undergoing sterilization and even other patients undertaking infertility treatment by assisted* reproduction techniques.

Pregnancy rates after donation are equivalent to those achieved with standard IVF and the pregnancies are not associated with increased problems, even though the fetus is genetically 100% 'foreign'. Like any other procedure which involves handling of gametes* or embryos*, egg donation in the UK may only be performed in clinics licensed by the HFEA*. As there is a severe shortage of donor eggs, the use of donor cards and alternative sources such as cadavers are being considered.

Egg donation raises complex medical, scientific, ethical, legal, social and psychological problems. Expert counselling* for both donors and recipients is essential and many cases are discussed by ethical* committees.

ejaculation: the discharge of semen* from the penis* during male orgasm. This occurs under the control of the autonomic nervous system. In the first phase, there is emptying of the contents of the epididymis*, the vas* deferens and seminal* vesicles into the prostatic urethra*. In the second phase, the bladder neck is occluded to prevent retrograde* ejaculation. In the

third phase, relaxation of the external urethral sphincter allows the rhythmic discharge of semen along the penile urethra.

ejaculation failure: this may occur in multiple sclerosis, spinal* cord injury, after retroperitoneal or pelvic surgery, as a result of certain drugs such as some antidepressants and antihypertensives or be of psychological origin. It can be overcome by certain movements of the patient which induce reflex ejaculation*, the use of an external penile* vibrator, rectal electro-ejaculation* and aspiration of the vas* deferens with retrieval of spermatozoa for AIH* or IVF*.

ejaculatory ducts: a pair of short straight ducts within the prostate* gland, through which spermatozoa*, stored in the ampulla of the vas* deferens, are propelled into the urethra* by the seminal* vesicle fluid during the first phase of ejaculation*. The ducts can be obstructed by small calculi, cysts* or inflammatory disease of the prostate or as a result of injury during bladder neck or prostate surgery.

If both ducts are obstructed, there is azoospermia* with a low volume of seminal* fluid which does not contain the fructose* normally secreted by the seminal* vesicles. This is identical to the semen from men with bilateral congenital absence of the vas deferens. If only one duct is occluded, there is a normal or reduced semen volume, which contains spermatozoa and fructose, but due to the presence of antisperm* antibodies, the sperm count and motility may be reduced. Obstruction of the ejaculatory ducts can be treated by endoscopic* surgery with a good chance of restoring fertility.

electro-ejaculation: treatment for ejaculation* failure: under general anaesthesia, electrodes are inserted through the anus to stimulate the seminal* vesicles through the anterior rectal wall. Semen* thus obtained is used for AIH*. This procedure has been used with considerable success in young men with paraplegia*.

embolism: the blockage of an artery* or vein* by an embolus* which causes interference with blood flow to sites beyond the place of lodgement. Serious loss of function may follow, especially if the embolus is large and lodged in the brain, lungs or major arteries. Treatment is with anticoagulant drugs to dissolve the blood clot or surgery (embolectomy).

embolus: a plug, commonly a blood clot, but which may also consist of other material such as air, fat or amniotic fluid. Emboli arise in the internal lining of arteries or veins, in the chambers of a poorly functioning heart, or may enter the circulation as result of trauma such as fracture of a bone. Deep vein thrombosis* in the calf is the commonest cause of embolus formation; this occurs particularly after surgery or confinement to bed for other reasons and is the main cause for the introduction of early mobilization after surgery or delivery.

embryo: the product of fertilization of an oocyte. A normal embryo, produced by the fertilization of an oocyte by one spermatozoon, is diploid* with a balanced complement of maternal and paternal chromosomes*. It will progress, by cleavage*, to the 2, 4, 8, 16 cell stages, become a morula* and finally, as the blastocyst*, implants into the uterine decidua* (Fig. 7).

In IVF*, embryos are produced by mixing together spermatozoa and oocytes. The embryos thus formed usually undergo cleavage* and are graded according to their appearance. The best quality embryos are transferred to the recipient's uterus or frozen (see cryopreservation). The grading methods used are subjective and normal pregnancies can still result from apparently poor quality embryos.

Genetically abnormal embryos may result from polyspermic* fertilization, parthenogenetically * activated cleavage*, an abnormal response of the oocyte to the penetrating spermatozoon or a genetic anomaly in either gamete*. In humans these mostly fail to implant or miscarry* at an early stage. Androgenetic embryos are those where the female genetic complement has been lost and only sperm-derived chromosomes remain. This is believed to be one mechanism by which hydatidiform* moles are formed.

In humans, the term embryo is applied to the conceptus from fertilization* until about the tenth week of gestation when most of the organs are developed and the embryo becomes a fetus.

embryo transfer (ET): the stage in IVF* when one or more embryos*, created

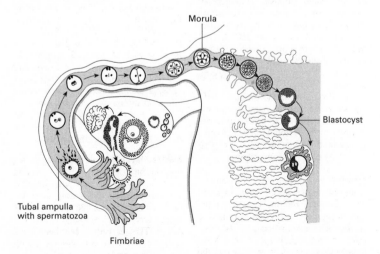

Fig. 7. Embryo development. Illustration showing ovulation, fertilization in the tubal ampulla, pronucleate stage, cleavage, morula and blastocyst stages, transport of the embryo to the uterus and implantation of the blastocyst.

in vitro, are transferred into the uterine* cavity by means of a specially designed catheter, passed through the cervical* canal.

embryonic genome activation: the point at which the developing embryo initiates transcription* from its own chromosomes*. Until this time, control of fertilization* and early cleavage* has been pre-programmed, relying upon maternal transcripts* formed during oocyte* development. In humans, embryonic genome activation occurs between the 4 and 8 cell stages of embryonic growth.

embryonic stem cells: see stem cells.

emergency contraception: see contraception.

endocrine gland: a ductless gland (e.g. pituitary*, thyroid*, ovary*, testis*) which secretes hormones* to targeted end organs via the bloodstream. Endocrine glands are usually under the control of stimulatory or inhibitory factors. Under- or over-activity can lead to life-threatening conditions.

endometrioma: a solitary deposit of endometriosis*; this can occur virtually anywhere in the body, typically in the ovaries* forming chocolate* cysts*. Other sites include lungs, liver, brain and scars after operations on the uterus.

endometriosis: the presence of endometrial cells* at sites other than the lining of the uterus*. This is a very common condition. The principal route of spread is by retrograde menstruation through the Fallopian* tubes with subsequent implantation of the endometrial deposits on peritoneal surfaces, especially the pelvic peritoneum, the ovaries, bowel or bladder. Spread may also occur through the uterine blood vessels or lymphatics with resultant implants at distant sites (e.g. the pleura). Spread by direct extension affects mainly the cornual* end of the tube and the uterine musculature (see adenomyosis, salpingitis isthmica nodosa). Spread can also follow delivery with implants in the vagina* or perineum* and can occur after uterine surgery with implants in the scar.

The ectopic endometrial tissue responds to the cyclical changes of the ovarian hormones and thus bleeding (menstruation*) occurs at the site of implantation, but the blood cannot escape. Implants can thus increase in size and this varies from microscopic deposits to others several centimetres in diameter. The repeated bleeds can cause pain, dysmenorrhoea* and deep dyspareunia* as well as generalized pelvic tenderness. Adhesions* may form as a result of the bleeding and scarring. Ovarian and pelvic endometriosis may be suspected from the patient's history and the findings on vaginal examination, but laparoscopy* is usually performed to make the definite diagnosis and determine the extent of the condition.

Views vary on the relation of minor degrees of endometriosis to infertility: much recent research suggests that mild endometriosis does not 'cause' infertility, but women with endometriosis do have a lower cumulative* conception rate than women with no endometriosis. In the more severe cases, adhesions* around the Fallopian* tubes and ovaries interfere with ovum* pick-up and transport, and ovarian chocolate* cysts may interfere with ovulation*. Some cases of endometriosis are entirely symptomless and only diagnosed at laparoscopy performed for unexplained* infertility or other causes.

Medical treatment of endometriosis should only be offered to women with symptoms such as pain, who are not trying to conceive; it has not been shown to improve fertility rates. Drugs used to treat endometriosis suppress ovulation and menstruation, thus allowing the disease to regress. They include the continuous use of high dose oestrogens* and/or progestogens*, danazol* or GnRH* analogues which suppress pituitary secretion of FSH* and LH*. All these treatments prevent conception. For women wishing to conceive, conservative surgical treatment, usually laparoscopic*, includes diathermy or laser* vaporization of the endometriosis deposits and adhesiolysis*. Superovulation* and intra-uterine* insemination is a valuable form of treatment, moving on to IVF* if this fails. IVF* should be offered straight away to women with dense, widespread adhesions which are not amenable to, or recur after, surgery. Radical surgery with removal of the uterus and ovaries may be necessary in older patients with advanced disease.

endometritis: inflammation of the endometrial* lining of the uterus*.

Acute endometritis is usually the result of infection ascending from the lower genital tract following delivery, miscarriage* or termination of pregnancy. Retained* products of conception encourage infection. Other causes include sexually* transmitted diseases such as chlamydia* or gonorrhoea*. Transluminal spread to the Fallopian* tubes may occur, causing tubal damage and subsequent subfertility. Symptoms may include fever, malaise, offensive vaginal discharge, irregular vaginal bleeding, pelvic pain and symptoms referable to pelvic peritonitis.

Puerperal endometritis (i.e. after delivery, miscarriage or termination) is a common cause of puerperal pyrexia and used to be the major cause of maternal mortality*. Modern obstetric techniques are geared to its prevention; prompt diagnosis and treatment with antibiotics are the basis of treatment.

Chronic endometritis can be due to tuberculosis* (which is blood-borne to the tubes from where there is direct spread to the uterus), submucous fibroids* or polyps, foreign bodies (IUCDs*), or ascending infection from chronic cervicitis*. Symptoms include offensive vaginal discharge, heavy menstrual losses and infertility. Diagnosis is by endometrial sampling or curettage* and treatment directed towards elimination of the particular cause.

endometrium: the layer of cells (mucosa) which lines the uterine* cavity (Fig. 26). These are mainly columnar epithelial cells which line the endometrial glands that course through the mucosa, extend down to the muscle of the uterus, and have a secretory function.

The cells which constitute this glandular lining are under the influence of the ovarian hormones* and progress through different phases during the menstrual* cycle. From the end of menstruation* until ovulation*, under the influence of oestrogens*, the endometrium is repaired and enters the proliferative phase during which it becomes thicker and the glands grow deeper. In the second half of the cycle, after ovulation*, under the influence of progesterone*, the endometrium enters its secretory phase during which there is a greatly increased blood flow and further glandular growth, now with marked secretory activity. If conception* occurs, the endometrium becomes the decidua* where the blastocyst* implants* and produces hCG* which stimulates the corpus* luteum to continue to secrete progesterone and prevent menstruation. If conception does not occur, oestrogen and progesterone production in the ovary declines, the hormonal support for the developed endometrium is withdrawn and the whole layer is shed in the process known as menstruation*. The menstrual loss thus consists of endometrial glands and secretions as well as blood.

The thickness of the endometrium can be measured by ultrasound* with a good correlation between its depth and functional activity. Endometrial biopsy is the removal of small strips of endometrium by curettage* or vacuum sampling. The specimens are submitted for histopathology to determine the hormonal status and detect any inflammatory or neoplastic changes.

endosalpinx: the mucous membrane lining the lumen of the Fallopian* tube.

endoscopy: the use of rigid or flexible tubes with a cold light source transmitting illumination via bundles of glass fibres to visualize interior parts of the body. The laparoscope* and hysteroscope* are the endoscopes most widely used by gynaecologists in the investigation and treatment of infertility. Endoscopes are also commonly used in other branches of medicine or surgery to view the inside of the bladder, stomach, bowel, bronchi and joints. Cameras are usually attached to the endoscopes to transmit images to video screens so that all theatre personnel, and not just the surgeon alone, can see and also so that permanent records can be kept.

Originally used for diagnosis only, endoscopy has now become the vehicle for minimal access surgery.

enucleation: the removal of the nuclear DNA* from a cell*. This is performed by micromanipulation*. In experimental embryology, oocytes* may be enucleated to allow them to act as host cells for a donated nucleus*, e.g. from a blastomere* as in cloning*. Enucleation of human oocytes is illegal in the UK.

enzyme: a protein* which catalyses a chemical reaction in a biological system. Most enzymes are highly specific, interacting with only a single or small range of related substances.

epididymis (Figs. 15, 25): the long, elaborately coiled tubule attached to the posterior aspect of the testis*, conveying spermatozoa* from the efferent ducts to the vas* deferens. The epididymis is divided into three parts: the head (caput) which consists mainly of efferent ducts before they unite to become the long coiled tubule of the body (corpus), and the wider tail (cauda) where sperms are stored prior to ejaculation. During their passage through the epididymis, the spermatozoa mature due to surface membrane changes and progressively gain motility and the ability to fertilize.

epididymitis: inflammation of the epididymis*, usually due, in younger men, to sexually* transmitted diseases. Chlamydia* has replaced gonorrhoea* as the commonest cause, and if the testis is also inflamed, the condition is known as epididymo-orchitis. This can be a very painful condition, but can also occur in a milder or silent form, and, if transmitted to the female partner by intercourse, may lead to pelvic* inflammatory disease (PID) with its sequelae. Similarly in the male partner, epididymitis can lead to scarring of the epididymis, which, if bilateral, may cause obstructive azoospermia*, and if unilateral, is a cause of antisperm* antibodies and oligozoospermia*. In older men, epididymitis can be associated with prostatic disease.

epididymo-vasostomy: a surgical anastomosis* between the vas* deferens and the epididymis*, carried out to bypass an obstruction of the epididymis in obstructive* azoospermia.

epididymal sperm aspiration (Fig. 24): a surgical procedure to retrieve spermatozoa* from the epididymis* in obstructive* azoospermia, either by micro-surgical epididymal sperm aspiration (MESA), usually performed under general anaesthesia, or by percutaneous epididymal sperm aspiration (PESA) which can be conveniently carried out under local anaesthesia.

epithelium: the tissues which line the outside of the body (the skin), the internal organs, blood vessels etc. Epithelial linings may be a thin, single cell layer or thick, multiple cell layers (stratified). The cells are subspecialized with, for example, squamous (flat, thin) and keratinized (tougher) cells protecting the skin, tall columnar cells lining the glands with special secretory functions and ciliated* cells lining the Fallopian* tubes with a role in gamete* transport.

equatorial segment: also known as the acrosomal collar (Fig. 23). An area in the sperm head with functions in the acrosome* reaction and the fusion of a spermatozoon* and oocyte*.

erection: increase in size and rigidity of the penis* (and to a lesser extent the clitoris*), achieved by the retention of blood in the sponge-like corpora* cavernosa. These changes are part of sexual arousal and, in the male, a necessary precursor to intercourse. They are under the control of the autonomic nervous system. Erection failure may be due to degenerative changes in the nerve fibres (common in diabetic males), Peyronie's* disease (fibrosis of the penis), or a side effect of various drugs; it is also associated with arteriosclerosis, hyperprolactinaemia*, testosterone* deficiency or psycho-sexual and marital problems. (See impotence.)

erythroblastosis: see haemolytic disease of the newborn.

Este's operation: the transplantation of ovarian tissue with a vascular pedicle into the upper uterine cavity. This operation used to be performed to treat irreparable tubal damage. The success rate was very low and the procedure has been abandoned in favour of IVF*.

ethinyl oestradiol: the synthetic form of oestradiol* used in the contraceptive* pill and in the treatment of some gynaecological disorders. The ethinyl group prevents metabolism in the gut and thus allows oral administration. Metabolism by the liver, however, can occasionally lead to hypertension* and coagulation changes.

ethics: the branch of philosophy concerned with human conduct. Medical ethics are concerned with the moral principles which govern medical practice. These principles include respect for patients' autonomy, benefiting patients, refraining from harming them, and observing justice and honesty in dealing with them. Advances in technology, e.g. assisted reproduction techniques, life support mechanisms and the need for allocation of scarce resources, can raise complex dilemmas of conflict between the rights of the individual and the needs of society. The obligations of health workers under these circumstances may be difficult to define.

Ethical committees have been set up in hospitals to advise on good practice and regulate research and most assisted reproduction clinics have such a committee. In the UK, fertility clinics which handle or store gametes* or embryos* are controlled and regulated by the HFEA* and their local ethical committees advise on research projects and controversial patient issues such as oocyte* and sperm* donation and surrogacy*.

eugenics: the use of science to attempt to improve the genetic* fitness of humans. Eugenics sank into disrepute during the 1930s and 1940s as a result of horror of the practices perpetrated by Nazi Germany and the forcible sterilization of immigrants and people of low intelligence in the USA and other countries. Since the Second World War emphasis has increasingly shifted towards enabling people to make their own reproductive decisions. Genetic* counselling can play an important role in this.

external cervical os (Fig. 26): the opening of the lower end of the cervical canal into the vagina*. The external os is circular or oval and small in women who have not given birth and larger, usually with a transverse slit, in women who have. (See also cervix.)

extra-uterine pregnancy (*syn.* ectopic pregnancy): the establishment of a pregnancy in sites other than the uterine* cavity. The commonest site is in the lumen of the Fallopian* tube which is too small to accommodate the enlarging gestational* sac, so that either tubal abortion or tubal rupture result. Ovarian ectopic pregnancy is rare. Very occasionally an extra-uterine pregnancy implants in a less confined site in the peritoneal cavity and may progress to fetal viability (advanced extra-uterine pregnancy: see abdominal pregnancy).

Ectopic pregnancies are an important cause of maternal morbidity and mortality*. There is currently no evidence that extra-uterine pregnancies can be relocated to the uterus and remain viable. The chances of having an extra-uterine pregnancy are increased in women with prolonged infertility, or with a past history of pelvic* inflammatory disease, sterilization*, previous extra-uterine pregnancy or tubal surgery, as well as in those using an intra-uterine* contraceptive device (IUCD) or undergoing IVF* treatment.

Salpingectomy* (surgical excision of the affected tube) used to be the standard treatment for tubal pregnancy. Recently, earlier diagnosis, before tubal abortion or rupture occurs, by the use of ultrasound* scans and quantitative hormonal pregnancy* tests (β subunit of hCG), has led to laparoscopic or medical treatment modalities which preserve the tube.

F

Fallopian tube (*syn.* oviduct Figs. 8, 26): one of the two long, thin, mobile, canalized structures which run outwards from the upper angle of the uterus* towards the ovary. Each tube is about 10 cm long and consists of the interstitial part which runs through the uterine musculature, a narrow isthmus*, wider ampulla* and the infundibulum* (abdominal ostium), shaped like a trumpet, which opens into the peritoneal cavity. This opening is surrounded by the fimbriae*, slender tentacle-like projections which play an important part in the ovum* pick-up mechanism. The lumen of the tube communicates via the uterine* cavity with the lower genital tract and via the abdominal ostium with the peritoneal cavity and can therefore be a pathway for the spread of ascending infection. The wall of the tube is muscular and with its peristaltic contractions plays a role in the passage of oocytes* and spermatozoa* through the genital tract. The inner lining (endosalpinx*) has many ciliated* cells which set up currents which also contribute to the ovum pick-up mechanism and the transport of the gametes*.

The functions of the tube relate to sperm transport, ovum pick-up, fertilization* (which occurs in the ampulla), nutrition and shelter for the developing zygote*, and its delivery into the uterine cavity at precisely the right time for implantation* five to seven days after ovulation*.

The tubes are a common site of infection (see salpingitis) which is usually bilateral and may cause adhesions* and scarring in the endosalpinx* predisposing to tubal pregnancy (see extra-uterine pregnancy). More extensive disease can cause blockage which occurs often at the utero–tubal junction, occasionally in the mid-tube, but most frequently at the abdominal ostium (see hydrosalpinx).

A tubal factor is present in more than 20% of women complaining of infertility. There are wide variations in this incidence in different ethnic groups, depending on environmental

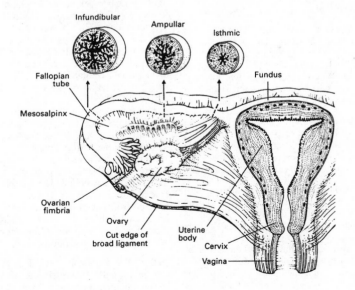

Fig. 8. The Fallopian tube and its relation to the ovary, broad ligment and uterus.

circumstances. The investigation of tubal patency and function is thus a routine part of infertility investigations and may include tubal* insufflation, hystero-salpingography*, laparoscopy*, falloposcopy* and salpingoscopy*.

falloposcopy: the transcervical cannulation and visual inspection of the lumen of the Fallopian* tube by a small fibre-optic* endoscope* (falloposcope), passed through the uterine* cavity via a hysteroscope* or under ultrasound* guidance. The procedure permits assessment of the endosalpinx* in patients suspected of having tubal infertility and thus makes possible better selection of patients for tubal surgery. In addition it can sometimes clear a blockage caused by mucus plugs at the utero–tubal* junction, and its role in the diagnosis and management of tubal pregnancy is currently being investigated.

familial: running in families. This usually means that a condition (e.g. a disease) has a genetic* component. However, it may simply be that the condition is the result of a common environment. For example, the tendency to speak French runs in families, but is not genetically inherited.

family planning: see contraception.

fecundity: a measure of the ability to produce offspring. This declines markedly with advancing maternal age*. The fecundability rate is the monthly probability of pregnancy when the opportunity for conception* exists (see also cumulative conception rate).

feeder layer: a culture of cells* on which another type of cell is incubated *in vitro*. The feeder layer may support the survival or function of the additional cultured cells. (See co-culture.)

ferning: the pattern resembling fern leaves observed when cervical* mucus is dried, allowed to crystallize, and inspected under the microscope. This is seen when the mucus becomes more profuse and fluid just before ovulation*, under the influence of oestrogens*, and thus is a favourable sign in the assessment of cervical mucus quality.

fertile period: the time in the menstrual* cycle when conception* is possible. This is usually just before, during or immediately after ovulation*, but the duration of the fertile period ultimately depends on the length of time the oocyte and sperm can survive in the genital tract. In a regular 28 days cycle, the fertile time is between days 10 and 14 and is usually marked by the appearance of a thin, oestrogenic* cervical* mucus at the external cervical os. Timed* intercourse is the attempt to use the fertile period either to enhance the chance of conception or to avoid conception. (See also basal body temperature.)

fertilization (Fig. 9): the process by which the male and female gametes* unite to form a zygote*. This begins when the spermatozoon* first contacts the oolemma* (the oocyte surface membrane) and lasts until the genetic material of sperm and oocyte* have mixed and reduplicated as the zygote* initiates its first division into two cells. *In vivo*, fertilization occurs in the Fallopian* tube, usually within one day of ovulation*, and is completed in approximately 24 hours. (See also *in vitro* fertilization.)

fertility: this term relates to the number of offspring born, expressed in relation to both population groups and individuals. In modern societies, women's fertility does not reach its maximum theoretical potential. Fertility declines with age* and is also influenced by duration of lactation*, contraception*, miscarriage*, termination of pregnancy and other social factors.

The fertility rate is the number of live births per 1000 female population of child bearing age. There are wide variations in the fertility rate in different countries and at different times in a country's development or history (e.g. the post-war baby boom). The age specific fertility rate reflects women's declining fertility with advancing years, but is also influenced by factors such as the age of first trying for a pregnancy and the use of contraception.

fetal alcohol syndrome: fetal damage can be caused by excessive alcohol consumption in pregnancy. Typically the infants exhibit varying degrees of

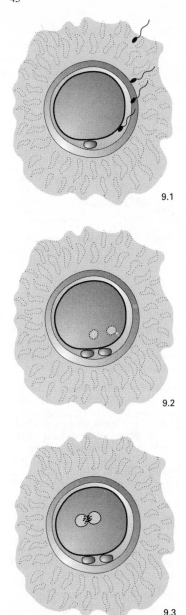

Fig. **9**. Fertilization.

9.1. The fertilizing sperm swims through the corona radiata cells, binds to the outside of the zona pellucida and then passes through it by means of swimming power and enzyme activity. Inside the zona pellucida, it binds with the oolemma and becomes immotile.

9.2. The sperm is absorbed into the oocyte, which becomes activated, releasing the second polar body and cortical granules into the perivitelline space. The sperm head decondenses and begins to form a pronucleus.

9.3. The sperm and the remaining oocyte chromatids form a pronucleus each. These migrate to the centre of the oocyte where the two pronuclei abut. The pronuclear membranes subsequently disintegrate, allowing the parental genetic contributions to mingle before progressing to the first mitotic (cleavage) division.

9.1

9.2

9.3

children lose the characteristic facial appearance, but they never attain normal height or intellectual function.

fetal reduction: an operative procedure to change an unwanted high order multiple* pregnancy (possibly the result of ovarian* stimulation) to a singleton or twin pregnancy and thus avoid the risks of extreme prematurity. The procedure may also be used in twin pregnancies if one of the twins is diagnosed, antenatally, to have a serious congenital abnormality. The technique employed is to inject potassium chloride into the fetal heart via a transvaginal or transabdominal approach and under ultra-sound* guidance. Possible complications include growth retardation of the surviving fetus(es), miscarriage* or premature delivery. The terms of the Abortion Act (1967) apply.

fetus: the offspring from the end of its embryonic stage until birth.

fibre-optics: flexible glass fibre cables, used to conduct brilliant 'cold light' illumination from an external light source into various body cavities. They form the basis of all modern endoscopy*.

fibroid (*syn*. fibromyoma, leiomyoma, myoma: Fig. 10): a benign encapsulated tumour arising from uterine*

mental retardation. At birth, they are underweight with small heads, eyes and lower jaws, upturned nose tips and long upper lips; they may be jittery or lethargic, with disturbed sleep patterns, failure to thrive and are liable to infections. By the age of five years, some

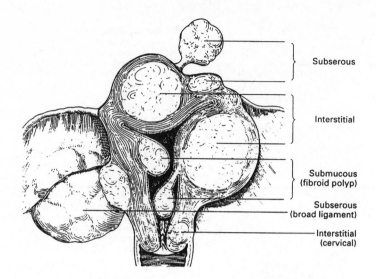

Fig. **10**. The sites of uterine fibroids.

muscle fibres. Fibroids are the commonest of all pelvic tumours, often multiple, and vary enormously in size. They occur more frequently in women over 30.

Fibroids may be subserous, i.e. on the outer surface of the uterus, with no effect on fertility; intra-mural, i.e. contained in the uterine musculature, in which case they may enlarge or distort the uterine cavity and/or cervical canal and may cause heavy menstruation, infertility or miscarriage*; or submucous, i.e. projecting into the uterine cavity, in which case they may cause heavy and/or irregular bleeding and prevent implantation* of an embryo.

Treatment, indicated if the fibroids cause significant symptoms or reach large size, is surgical. Myomectomy* is performed in women wishing to preserve their reproductive function. Submucous fibroids can be resected through the hysteroscope*. Hysterectomy* is commonly performed in older women, usually with preservation of the ovaries if they are not yet menopausal*.

fibrosis: the sequel of inflammatory or irritative processes (especially if repeated) involving muscle or other tissues. Thickening and scarring of the affected tissue may interfere with function as in the thickened, rigid Fallopian* tubes seen after repeated episodes of salpingitis*.

filial: of a son or daughter. So, geneticists refer to the F_1 (i.e. 1st filial) generation, meaning the offspring that result from a cross between two individuals. Strictly, these two individuals should each be homozygous* for the gene* in question. The term is more usually used in agriculture and biological research than in human genetics.

fimbria ovarica: one of the tubal fimbriae* which is longer than the others and extends to the tubal pole of the ovary. It enables the fimbriated end of the tube to sweep over the ovarian surface, an essential part of the ovum* pick-up mechanism.

fimbriae (Fig. 8): the elongated slender folds of mucous membrane arranged as a fringe around the abdominal ostium* of the Fallopian* tubes and richly lined with ciliated* cells. There are 10 to 15 fimbriae on each infundibulum*, each 10 to 15 mm long. At the time of ovulation* the fimbriae sweep over the ovarian surface and thus take part in the ovum* pick-up mechanism.

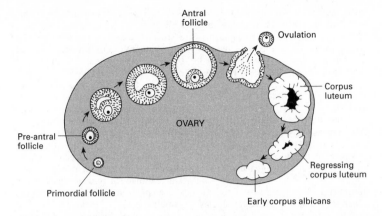

Fig. 11. Follicle development. Development of an ovarian follicle, proceeding to ovulation and subsequent corpus luteum formation.

Adhesions* restricting the mobility of the fimbriated end of the tube are a common cause of tubal infertility. In complete occlusion of the abdominal end of the tube, the fimbriae are withdrawn into the infundibulum and cannot be seen at laparoscopy (see hydrosalpinx, salpingostomy). Less severe degrees of fimbrial damage are agglutination or phimosis* (see fimbrioplasty).

fimbrioplasty: the surgical procedure to reconstruct the abdominal* ostium when it is partially occluded (see fimbriae, phimosis). Such occlusion is usually accompanied by peri-tubal adhesions*, and adhesiolysis* has to be performed first. Fimbrioplasty is performed either by open abdominal surgery or by laparoscopy*.

FISH (fluorescence *in situ* hybridization): a technique which combines microscopy with nucleic* acid probes to localize specific DNA* sequences. Probes complementary to a particular DNA sequence are labelled by incorporating individual bases modified to incorporate a radioactive atom or an epitope (the particular part of an antigen* molecule to which the corresponding antibody* binds). The probe only binds specifically to RNA or DNA with the particular sequence under study and elucidates its location. The technique can be used in embryo pre-implantation* diagnosis and also in research to determine whether a particular gene* is being transcribed* or for the location of specific genes on chromosomes* (see transcription).

Fisher's Exact Test (for contingency* tables): a non-parametric* test which is an alternative to the very popular Chi-squared* test, and which should be used when the expected frequencies in the cells are small (say < 5). It is a computer intensive test, for which tables have now been published for a limited range of frequencies. Algorithms are also available to carry out the test. The very laborious calculations involve computing the probabilities of various table configurations, under the assumption of independence of the marginal classifications.

Fitz-Hugh Curtis syndrome: inflammation of the liver producing right- sided upper abdominal pain, usually secondary to pelvic infection caused by *Chlamydia*.

folic acid: a B group vitamin which is utilized in DNA* synthesis. Deficiency can lead to defective cell proliferation. Pregnant women have increased folic acid requirements for the normal development of the placenta* and fetus*. Women who give birth to babies with neural* tube defects (see anencephaly, spina bifida) have lower levels of intracellular folic acid than women whose babies are normal. Oral daily intake of small doses of folic acid in very early pregnancy, ideally started before conception* or on discontinuing contraception*, reduces the incidence of recurrence of neural tube defects in women with a previously affected baby; it has been shown that pre-conceptual use is also beneficial in women who have not previously had an affected baby.

Methotrexate*, a folic acid antagonist, arrests development of early pregnancies and can be used in the conservative management of unruptured tubal extra-uterine* pregnancy.

follicle (Fig. 11): the group of cells in which the oocyte* is situated. Follicles first form in the female fetus during the fourth month of gestation, when developing germ* cells become surrounded by a small group of flattened somatic ovarian cells. These primordial* follicles are the smallest, about 0.03 mm in diameter, and about 7 million are formed initially. By the time of birth, their number has declined to about 2 million. After puberty*, a constant small proportion of follicles start growing each day but only about 400 will ever release a mature oocyte; a far greater number never mature and finally undergo atresia*. The menopause* occurs when the reserve of oocytes has been depleted to less than about 1000.

Initially follicular growth is independent of gonadotrophins*, but in larger follicles it is regulated by the secretion of FSH* and LH*. Growing follicles pass through various stages of development, from primordial to primary (with a single layer of cuboidal granulosa* cells), secondary (with two layers of granulosa cells), pre-antral (with several layers of granulosa cells), antral (with several layers of granulosa cells and a fluid-filled cavity called an antrum*) and pre-ovulatory, known as the Graafian* follicle, (with an enlarged fluid filled antrum and the oocyte at the side of the follicle, surrounded by cumulus* and corona* cells). As they grow, follicles become surrounded by specialized theca* cells which are separated from the granulosa cells by a basement membrane. The theca is broadly divided into two areas: theca interna and theca externa: the latter contains blood vessels, nerves

and muscle fibres which hold the follicle in shape and, in some species, assist in ovulation*. The theca interna and granulosa cells produce steroid* hormones from which oestradiol* and progesterone* are derived.

The leading follicle can reach 20 mm or more in diameter, and when it ruptures (ovulation) the oocyte is released to the outer surface of the ovary from where it may be picked up by the tubal fimbriae* and transported towards the uterus. Follicles occasionally persist and enlarge to form ovarian cysts*. This can happen spontaneously but is also a common side effect of ovarian* stimulation.

For clinical assessment, follicular size is measured by ultrasound*, and oestradiol* concentrations may be used as an index of function. For superovulation (ovarian* stimulation), as in an IVF* treatment cycle, large doses of FSH* are administered so that some or all of the available follicles are stimulated to grow.

follicular fluid: this fluid is found in the antrum* of a developing follicle*. It is primarily an exudate of blood plasma, filtered through the follicle's basement membrane and granulosa layers, but is also highly conditioned by the granulosa* cells adjacent to the cavity which produce numerous substances including large amounts of steroids*, proteins*, enzymes* and low molecular weight compounds. The types and quantities of the compounds in follicular fluid vary as the follicle enlarges and matures.

The follicular fluid probably acts as a fluid medium for transporting the oocyte* out of the follicle at ovulation*. Follicular fluid is aspirated from the follicles when oocytes are collected for assisted* reproduction procedures. It is examined microscopically for the presence of an oocyte and may be analysed chemically for various products which may reflect the health of the follicle at the time of collection.

follicular phase: the period of development in which the dominant follicle* (with its oocyte* and theca and granulosa cells*) grows to become a fully formed Graafian* follicle,

responsive to the pre-ovulatory LH*
surge. The follicular phase usually lasts
14 days.

follicle stimulating hormone (FSH): one
of the two gonadotrophins* produced
by the pituitary* gland under the influence of GnRH*. In women it stimulates the growth and differentiation of
the granulosa* cells in the developing
follicle* and their role in converting
androgens* to oestradiol*. The serum
FSH concentration rises in the menopause and can be used as a diagnostic
indicator of its onset.

In men, FSH, acting via the Sertoli*
cells in the seminiferous* tubules, initiates spermatogenesis* by the testis*.
If there is absent (anorchia) or deficient
spermatogenesis, the FSH concentration is usually raised.

fornix: *pl.* fornices (Fig. 26): the regions of the vaginal* vault in relation to
the cervix* as it projects into the upper
vagina, divided into an anterior, a posterior and two lateral fornices. During
vaginal examination, structures such
as the Fallopian* tubes and ovaries*
are palpated through the fornices. The
lateral fornices are punctured during
vaginal oocyte* collection for IVF*.

fourchette (Fig. 27): the area where the
two labia* minora meet and fuse posteriorly, thus forming the lower border
of the vaginal entrance. In lacerations
sustained during childbirth, this is the
first structure to be injured.

fragile-X syndrome: a sex-linked* genetic* disorder, occurring mainly in
males, and causing mental retardation
of varying degree. Affected men may
have elongated faces with large fore-
heads and enlarged testes, but these
features are not always present. The
prevalence of fragile-X syndrome is
about 1 in 1000 males and this is

probably the second commonest cause
of mental retardation, after Down's*
syndrome. As opposed to Down's syndrome, the older a woman is, the less
likely she is to have a son with fragile-
X syndrome.

freezing: see cryopreservation.

free radicals: molecules which are
chemically unstable, having a tendency
to form highly reactive oxidants, such
as superoxides. Production of free radicals is encouraged by cellular damage.
Free radicals damage cell membranes
and may affect processes such as fertilization* and cell division. Naturally
occurring enzymes, such as superoxide
dismutase, scavenge the free radicals
in vivo. These enzymes are not present
in vitro unless they have been specifically added to the medium: therefore
efforts to avoid damage to oocytes,
spermatozoa and embryos from degen-
erating cells are important, in order
to ensure that unnecessary damage to
membranes is avoided.

Concentrations of free radicals (reactive* oxygen species) are raised in
the semen* of many subfertile men,
and may indicate subclinical infection.

frigidity: failure of sexual arousal. The
term is usually applied to women only.
It is not to be confused with failure
to achieve orgasm which may occur
despite full arousal. Frigidity is not in
itself an infertility factor, except when
associated with decreased sexual activity or vaginismus*.

fructose: a sugar normally produced
by the seminal* vesicles and present in
seminal* plasma. It provides energy for
the spermatozoa* and is essential for
their motility. It is absent when there
is ejaculatory* duct obstruction or congenital absence of the vas* deferens.

G

galactorrhoea: the secretion of milk from the breasts when there is no lactation*. Small amounts of milk can be expressed in normal women for varying lengths of time after the cessation of lactation. Galactorrhoea, especially if associated with amenorrhoea* or other menstrual irregularities, may be a side effect of certain drugs, e.g. antidepressants, or a sign of hormonal disorders such as hyperprolactinaemia*, thyroid* abnormalities and, ocasionally, polycystic* ovarian syndrome.

Galactorrhoea is rare in men and usually asociated with hyperprolactinaemia.

gamete: the male and female sex cells, i.e. the mature oocyte* and sperm* which are capable of combining together to form a new genetic individual. Gametes have half the usual chromosome* content (23), known as haploid*, having undergone meiosis* so that the combination of the male and female gametes at fertilization results in the formation of a zygote* with the normal number of 46 chromosomes, known as diploid*.

Gardnerella vaginalis: see bacterial vaginosis.

gender: classification of a person as male or female. Gender identity is the gender to which an individual considers him/herself to belong, and usually corresponds to the gender assigned at birth. Gender role is the behaviour society considers appropriate and expects from a male or female. Gender disorders may be related to the finding of ambiguous external genitalia at birth (e.g. adreno-genital* and testicular* feminization syndromes) or may be psychogenic (e.g. transvestites, transsexuals).

gene: a term used in several senses, but most easily thought of as the unit of inheritance. Some characteristics, for example whether a person has blood that is Rhesus positive or Rhesus negative, are determined by single genes. Other characteristics, for example natural hair colour, are determined by the actions of several genes. Most characteristics, for example height and personality, are determined jointly by the interaction of the environment and several genes.

An individual gene consists of several hundred bases (see DNA). It is the order of these chemical bases that uniquely determines the properties of genes. The genes themselves are codes for proteins*, each gene typically being responsible for the synthesis of a single protein. For example, our muscles contain a number of different proteins. Each muscle protein is coded for by a different gene.

Each of the normal cells in our body contains two copies of each gene (see diploid cell). One of these copies comes from the oocyte*; the other from the spermatozoon* which has succeeded in fertilizing that oocyte. Oocytes and spermatozoa (known as haploid* cells) have only one copy of each gene.

Humans have approximately 80 000 genes, each so small as to be virtually invisible, even with the electron microscope. Yet the smallest mistake in the structure of a gene may lead to an inherited disorder such as cystic* fibrosis or Huntingdon's* chorea.

gene disorder: a type of congenital* disorder in which the mistake is in a single gene*. For example, cystic* fibrosis and Duchenne* muscular dystrophy are example of gene disorders, whereas Down's* syndrome and Klinefelter's* syndrome are chromosomal* disorders which can be observed microscopically.

gene therapy: a procedure in which healthy genes* are given to patients in an attempt to cure a disease. The usual procedure is that copies of the healthy gene are obtained from a human donor and inserted into the genetic material of a bacterium*. The bacterium is then allowed to multiply, which it does very rapidly. The healthy human genes are then extracted from the bacteria using natural enzymes* and inserted into a vector such as a harmless virus*. The vector then carries these copies of the healthy human gene into certain of the cells of a diseased patient. Here the hope is that the copies of the healthy genes insert themselves into the person's genetic material and start to make the desired substances (often enzymes*) which the patient lacks.

Research into gene therapy is currently under way in several countries and is attempting to tackle a number of human diseases. For example, people with cystic* fibrosis have been given the healthy version of the cystic fibrosis gene, though it is too early to be confident that this approach offers significant therapeutic advantages.

Many ethical* committees have considered whether gene therapy should be allowed. Most have concluded that somatic gene therapy—in which changes are made to the normal body cells (i.e. diploid* cells)—is ethically acceptable, not really being very different from any medical procedure in which a person is given a substance, e.g. insulin, which they are unable to make for themselves. However, the same ethical committees have generally cautioned against germ-line gene therapy, at least for the time being. In germ-line gene therapy, changes are made not just to the genetic material of individuals, but—via alterations to the structure of the individual's spermatozoa* or oocytes*—to their descendants in perpetuity. Fears have been expressed that gene therapy might be used to alter people's personalities or intelligence. While this is unlikely, the technique does open up new possibilities and raises questions about how far humans should go in their exploitation of new medical technologies.

genetic counselling: a confidential service in which a counsellor* helps a person or a couple to make decisions about having children in the light of information about their genetic make-up. An example is a couple who have had a child with Down's* syndrome or sickle-cell* anaemia and want to know what the risks are that any future children they have may also be affected. A genetic counsellor will answer their questions and help them to explore all the medical and legal options available, which may include a termination if the woman is pregnant. A good genetic counsellor will do this in such a way that the person or couple understands what is going on and can make up their own mind(s) in the light of all the relevant, available information. (See also screening.)

genital herpes: a common infection caused by the herpes* simplex virus type 1 or 2. First attacks produce severe and painful genital ulceration and may or may not be followed by recurrences which in most cases are milder than the first attack. Early oral antiviral treatment dramatically reduces the severity of first attacks and may be used to suppress recurrences.

Transmission from mother to child may take place in labour and is most likely after a first attack in pregnancy. Such occurrence may be an indication for delivery by Caesarean* section. The risk to the fetus is reduced in recurrent attacks. Neonatal herpes is a severe and in some cases fatal disease. (See herpes.)

genital warts: see warts.

genome: all the genetic material (i.e. the DNA*) within the cells of an individual. The human genome contains approximately 80 000 genes*.

genome activation: the point at which the chromosomes* of spermatozoa* and oocytes* start to control the cell* by making proteins*, after the oocyte has been fertilized*. Fertilization* and the early events after fertilization are controlled by genetic messages programmed into the oocyte during its growth and maturation. The paternal chromosomes in the fertilizing sperm therefore do not take part in controlling these events.

The embryonic genome*, consisting of both oocyte and sperm chromosomes, probably takes over control of embryo development at the third cleavage* division (4–8 cells) in humans.

genotype: the genetic make-up of an individual, as opposed to his/her external appearance (the phenotype*).

German measles: see rubella.

germ cell: ancestral cell from which a specific cell type or range of related cells are formed: e.g. primordial germ cells form oocytes* or spermatozoa* and bone marrow germ cells produce all types of blood cells.

germinal epithelium: a thin layer of columnar epithelium* which covers the ovary*. This used to be considered as the site of production of primordial follicles*. These are now known to form in the cortex (outer zone) of the ovary in fetal life and the germinal epithelium is more correctly considered as only a surface epithelial layer. A similar situation exists in the testis*.

germinal vesicle: the characteristic conformation of the nucleus* of an immature oocyte* arrested in prophase I of meiosis*. The germinal vesicle nucleus has a pale, plain appearance, with usually a single large nucleolus. The oocyte may remain in this stage indefinitely, from its formation in the fetus until its maturation or atresia* at any time before the menopause*, sometimes for as long as 50 years. The first visible sign of impending maturation is often the movement of the germinal vesicle from the centre to the periphery of a fully grown oocyte.

gestational sac (Fig. 20): the pregnancy complex, consisting of membranes and amniotic* fluid and containing the fetus* and its placenta*. The sac may be 'empty', as diagnosed by ultrasound* scan, when no fetus has developed (see blighted ovum*) or 'disappearing' when a non-viable pregnancy (for example one of twins) is absorbed. The gestational sac is punctured when fluid is withdrawn at amniocentesis*.

GIFT: gamete intra-fallopian transfer. In this assisted* reproduction technique, oocytes* are collected (after ovarian* stimulation) by laparoscopy* or vaginal ultrasound directed aspiration. They are mixed with a prepared specimen of semen*, and introduced into the Fallopian* tube either laparoscopically or transvaginally. Fertilization* thus occurs in the tube (as opposed to in vitro* fertilization).

GIFT should only be performed if the tubes are both patent and healthy to avoid the risk of extra-uterine* pregnancy. The main indications for GIFT are unexplained* infertility and certain of the less severe types of male infertility. No licence from the HFEA* is required for GIFT unless donated spermatozoa are used. Some religious anthorities prefer GIFT to IVF because the former avoids extra-corporeal conception.

globozoospermia: a rare male fertility disorder where the acrosome* of the sperm head fails to develop. Spermatozoa are thus 'round' or 'marble-headed' and cannot fertilize, even in vitro. ICSI* with acrosomeless spermatozoa has resulted in pregnancies but at a lower success rate than ICSI with normally formed spermatozoa.

gonads: the testes* and ovaries* in which the gametes* are formed.

gonadal dysgenesis: genetically determined failure of the gonad* (testis or ovary) to produce germ* cells. Turner's* syndrome in the female and Klinefelter's* syndrome in the male are the commonest examples.

gonadotrophin releasing hormone (GnRH): also known as luteinizing hormone releasing hormone* (LHRH): this is a hypothalamic* factor, a decapeptide, which, after the onset of puberty*, regulates in a pulsatile manner the synthesis of gonadotrophins* (FSH and LH) by the pituitary* gland and their release into the circulation. GnRH itself is rapidly broken down and hardly detectable in the peripheral circulation. Production of GnRH is influenced by dietary habits, body weight, exercise, light and the blood levels of steroids* and other hormones. The amenorrhoea* often seen in anorexic* patients or in athletes is associated with reduced GnRH synthesis.

GnRH analogues (e.g. Buserelin*) are substances in which one or more of the amino* acids in GnRH are substituted by a different amino acid, to produce alterations in activity and binding to receptors. The agonist analogues bind to receptors of the gonadotrophins and release stored FSH and LH. Prolonged usage leads to reversible hypogonadotrophic* hypogonadism which is associated with low oestrogen* concentrations and anovulation*. This property leads to their use in shrinking fibroids*, in the treatment of endometriosis* and, in men, to control prostatic cancer by reducing testosterone* secretion. The analogues are used in fertility treatment to suppress the LH* surge and thus allow controlled ovarian* stimulation.

gonadotrophins: this term comprises follicle* stimulating hormone (FSH) and luteinizing* hormone (LH) produced by the pituitary* gland and human* chorionic gonadotrophin (hCG) produced by the placenta*.The pituitary gonadotrophins are produced in a pulsatile manner, with variations throughout the menstrual cycle, under the influence of hypothalamic GnRH*. They stimulate the growth and differentiation of follicles* and steroid* production from the ovarian granulosa* and theca* cells. Concentrations of pituitary gonadotrophins are very low before puberty* and in women with amenorrhoea* due to dysfunction of the hypothalamus* or pituitary gland, i.e. weight- or exercise-related amenorrhoea, Kallman's* syndrome, hyperprolactinaemia* and Sheehan's* syndrome.

In ovulatory cycles, FSH concentrations are relatively high during the follicular* phase, thus stimulating the development of the dominant follicle. The subsequent rise in oestradiol*, produced by the follicular granulosa cells, suppresses FSH, but, at a certain threshold, stimulates the surge of LH which initiates ovulation*. Both FSH and LH are suppressed in the luteal* phase by the high progesterone* levels.

Clomiphene* citrate increases the secretion of endogenous gonadotrophins: it is used to stimulate ovulation* in anovulatory* women, such as those with polycystic* ovarian syndrome. Around the time of the menopause*, gonadotrophin concentrations increase since oestrogen* secretion diminishes as follicles* become fewer in number and less responsive. Purified urine from post-menopausal women contains high levels of FSH and LH and is marketed as hMG* (human menopausal gonadotrophin). Administration of such a preparation during the early follicular phase can induce multiple follicular development prior to egg collection and IVF* (see

ovarian stimulation). Ovarian* hyperstimulation can be a serious side effect of gonadotrophin therapy.

In men, FSH and LH are the same hormones as in women, with similar actions on the testes* (LH used to be known as interstitial cell stimulating hormone). They are essential for spermatogenesis* and testosterone* secretion. Deficiency leads to hypogonadotrophic* hypogonadism; this usually responds well to treatment with gonadotrophins. The FSH concentration is grossly elevated in primary testicular failure and both FSH and LH concentrations are greatly elevated in men with testosterone deficiency due to hypogonadism*, e.g. Klinefelter's* syndrome.

Due to a world-wide shortage of human derived gonadotrophins, biosynthetic FSH and LH have been developed as the first line in treatment. (See recombinant DNA technology.)

gonorrhoea: a sexually* transmitted infection caused by a bacterium*, *Neisseria gonorrhoea*. The incubation period is 2 to 8 days.

In women, gonorrhoea can be asymptomatic, but more usually presents with urinary symptoms and a heavy muco-purulent discharge. The lower genital tract is the primary site of infection, but spread to the upper genital tract may cause pelvic* inflammatory disease and its sequelae of tubal infertility and extra-uterine* pregnancy.

In men, pain on passing urine and a muco-purulent penile discharge are the first symptoms, and the infection may spread to the prostate*, testes* (epididymo-orchitis*) and other parts of the body. Scarring of the tail of the epididymis* or the vas* deferens may lead to obstructive* azoospermia.

Antibiotics are effective treatment in early cases, but not once structural damage has occurred. Strains of *N. gonorrhoea* resistant to many antibiotics have evolved. Pregnant women with gonorrhoea may transmit the infection to their baby in labour, resulting in a severe eye infection, ophthalmia neonatorum, which, if untreated, leads to blindness.

Tracing and treating sexual contacts*, who may be symptom-free, is an essential part of the management.

goserelin: a GnRH* analogue, used as a depot injection for the treatment of endometriosis* and, in men, prostatic* cancer.

Graafian follicle: the large pre-ovulatory follicle*, named after de Graaf who also first described the seminiferous* tubules in the testis*.

granulosa cells: ovarian* somatic cells contained within the basement membrane of the follicle*. Different types of granulosa cells exist, e.g. mural—close to the basement membrane and theca* layers; antral—close to the antrum*; cumulus*—surrounding the oocyte but not in immediate contact with it and coronal*—in contact with the oocyte. Granulosa cells produce oestradiol* and other hormones.

granulosa lutein cell: see luteal cell.

gravid: adjective meaning to be in a state of pregnancy. Gravidity refers to the number of episodes of pregnancy a woman has had. A woman having her first pregnancy is referred to as gravida 1 or primigravida. The term should not be confused with parity which means having given birth. Thus a gravida 2, para 1 indicates a woman who has had two pregnancies, one resulting in the birth of a child and the other relating to a previous pregnancy which terminated in a miscarriage, or to a present on-going pregnancy. A multigravida is a woman who has had more than one pregnancy.

growth factors: proteins* which act through receptors to influence biological processes throughout the body including follicle* growth, oocyte* maturation, spermatogenesis* and steroid* biosynthesis. They form an integral part of the control mechanisms of all living cells and act as regulators of multiplication and/or differentiation of cells*. Numerous families of growth factors exist and examples include insulin-like growth factors, epidermal growth factors and transforming growth factors.

growth hormone: a hormone* produced in the anterior lobe of the pituitary* gland which regulates bodily growth and stimulates insulin-like growth* factor production by the liver. Deficiency in childhood is one of the causes of short stature. Excessive secretion before puberty causes gigantism, and in adults acromegaly*. The addition of growth hormone may be beneficial in the stimulation of unifollicular ovulation* in patients who show poor response to gonadotrophin*.

gynaecomastia: enlargement of the breasts in males which can be unilateral or bilateral. It can occur at puberty* as part of normal development. It is usually a side effect of certain drugs such as spironolactone (a diuretic), cimetidine (used for the treatment of gastric and duodenal ulcers) or anabolic steroids* (used for body building). It may be associated with thyroid* disease or Klinefelter's* syndrome and can also be caused by a prolactin-producing tumour of the pituitary* gland (see hyperprolactinaemia*). It may be the first symptom of testicular cancer, making further investigations mandatory.

H

habitual abortion: see recurrent miscarriage.

haematocoele: a collection of old blood, usually originating from bleeding from an extra-uterine* (tubal) pregnancy, sited in the pouch of Douglas*. The term is also applied to a collection of blood in the tunica* vaginalis of the testis* and may be a complication of percutaneous* epididymal sperm aspiration (PESA).

haematocolpos: distension of the vagina* by old menstrual blood which cannot escape due to an imperforate hymen*.

haematometra: distension of the uterine cavity by blood. This may be due to retention of menstrual blood which cannot escape (see haematocolpos, imperforate hymen) but can also be due to vaginal atresia* or cervical* stenosis.

haematuria: blood in the urine. This may be the result of infections, tumours, stones or other diseases of the urethra*, bladder, ureters or kidneys and requires full investigation in both men and women.

haemoglobinopathy: the group of recessively* inherited abnormalities of the globin chains of haemoglobin in the red blood cells. Normal adult haemoglobin contains both α haemoglobin and β haemoglobin. α thalassaemia is due to underproduction of α haemoglobin and β thalassaemia to underproduction of β haemoglobin. In these there are no abnormalities of haemoglobin structure. Abnormalities of structure are known as the variant haemoglobins of which the commonest is sickle*.

When a person has inherited only one abnormal gene*, or allele*, from one of the parents, there is no ill health and the person is heterozygous* and known as a 'carrier' or as having the 'trait'. When two abnormal genes are inherited, one from each parent, a serious disorder usually results, which is homozygous* if the same genes are inherited from both parents as in sickle*-cell anaemia or β thalassaemia* major. Screening* of women before conception* or at antenatal clinics can be performed by blood tests, haemoglobin electrophoresis and the sickle* test. Any women who is found to have a haemoglobinopathy (trait or disease) should be counselled and her partner invited for testing so that prenatal* diagnosis can be offered to couples at risk of having a child with a major haemoglobinopathy.

haemolytic disease of the new-born: this abnormality, formerly known as erythroblastosis, occurs when a woman has been immunized to a blood group which is present on the fetus' red blood cells. The IgG antibody* crosses the placenta* and causes haemolysis (destruction of red cells) in the fetus. The degree of haemolysis can vary from mild through moderate to so severe as to cause death from heart failure *in utero*.

The commonest cause of haemolytic disease of the new-born is immunization to Rh(D), known as Rhesus disease. Women who are Rhesus negative but carry a Rhesus positive (D) fetus (inherited from the Rhesus positive father) have usually been immunized in previous pregnancies or by small bleeds from the fetal into the maternal circulation in the present pregnancy. In the UK, a passive* immunization programme with anti-D has resulted in almost total disappearance of severe haemolytic disease of the new-born. However, babies occasionally still need treatment after birth ('exchange transfusion') or even with transfusion *in utero*. Antibody* screening of maternal serum is performed routinely in antenatal clinics to detect immunization to Rhesus and other antigens*.

haemophilia: a sex-linked*, inherited abnormality of Factor VIII in the blood clotting cascade. 30 to 40% of cases of haemophilia result from spontaneous new mutations* in the Factor VIII gene*. The abnormal gene is carried on one of the X chromosomes* and, therefore, through the female line. Females are, almost always, asymptomatic whilst their sons have a 1 in 2 risk of inheriting the abnormal gene, resulting in low Factor VIII levels and spontaneous prolonged bleeding. Treatment is by periodic intravenous infusions of Factor VIII concentrate.

Many patients were infected with viruses, including HIV* and hepatitis* B and C, prior to the introduction of screening blood donors for these viruses and the production of recombinant* products.

haemorrhagic disease of the new-born: this occurs as a result of immaturity of the liver in the new-born with low synthesis of various blood clotting factors and can give rise to life-threatening bleeding soon after delivery. Vitamin K is generally given to all babies at birth in order to promote production of these clotting factors and reduce the risk of bleeding.

haemospermia: the presence of blood in semen*. In men aged below 40 this is usually due to prostatitis* or other low grade infection of the genital tract. However in men over 40 a tumour of the bladder or other parts of the urogenital tract must be excluded.

hamster test (*syn.* hamster oocyte penetration test): a test of the fertilizing ability of human spermatozoa* by observing their penetration into zona*-free hamster eggs. Spermatozoa which are unable to enter the eggs are considered to be dysfunctional. The test is too elaborate and complicated for routine clinical work and has largely been superseded by other investigations and more recently by the development of treatments such as ICSI*.

haploid cell: a cell with only one set of chromosomes*. In humans, haploid cells contain 23 chromosomes*. Only the gametes* (oocytes and spermatozoa) are haploid. Almost all the other cells in a person are diploid* with 46 chromosomes.

hatching: the process by which the blastocyst* escapes from the zona* pellucida before implantation*. *In vitro*, hatching may occur on about day 7 of embryo development. Some embryos appear unable to hatch, possibly because the zona pellucida is too thick or has become hardened. It is not known whether blastocysts undergo the same hatching *in vivo*, where the uterine environment may soften or dissolve the zona pellucida (see assisted hatching). Assisted hatching before embryo* transfer may be used to promote implantation* after IVF*.

hepatitis: inflammation of the liver which may be caused by one of a number of viruses*.

Hepatitis A is transmitted by the faecal–oral route via contaminated food or water. It has a relatively short incubation period of three to five weeks, causes a short-lived illness with malaise and jaundice and is not associated with chronic liver disease.

Hepatitis B (formerly known as serum hepatitis) is transmitted by blood contact (including transfusion of infected blood products and intravenous drug usage) and by sexual contact, both heterosexual and homosexual. In the developing world, most infections are acquired during birth by the offspring of infected mothers (vertical transmission). There may be an acute illness, but the majority of patients are symptom-free. 1% of infected adults develop a severe and fatal illness (fulminant hepatitis) and 10 to 15% become chronic and infectious carriers of the virus; in neonates this figure rises to almost 100%. Some chronic carriers eventually develop cirrhosis and cancer of the liver. However, 85–90% of infected people clear the infection and develop protective antibody*.

The incubation period for hepatitis B is two to six months. All blood and tissue donors, including sperm and oocyte donors, are now screened for hepatitis B as are most patients undergoing assisted conception, especially IVF* and ICSI*. The carrier state is common throughout the world and presents special hazards to surgeons and other health professionals. Similarly, infected health professionals are a potential danger to their patients. Health care workers and others who are at risk of contact with infected blood or other secretions are now vaccinated against the infection. Treatment of chronic carriers with interferon is sometimes successful.

Hepatitis C (formerly known as non-A, non-B hepatitis) is also transmitted by blood contact; sexual and vertical transmission is frequent. The initial illness is usually mild but may be followed in an unknown proportion of cases by chronic liver disease. In the UK, blood and blood products have been screened for hepatitis C since 1989. In assisted conception units, both partners are usually tested before having treatment. Interferon treatment is currently being evaluated. The incidence of hepatitis B and C is hopefully decreasing as a result of the greater safety of blood and blood products, and other measures such as the issue of free needles to drug users and the use of condoms for 'safe sex'.

Hepatitis D occurs only in association with hepatitis B and increases the severity of the disease. Hepatitis E is transmitted by the faecal–oral route and is sometimes associated with hepatitis epidemics.

hermaphroditism: in true hermaphroditism there is failure of complete sexual differentiation into either male or female: affected individuals have both testicular* and ovarian* tissue with ambiguous external genitalia and a wide spectrum of genital tract disorders.

Pseudo-hermaphrodites have either ovaries or testes, but not both; however their sexual appearance is at variance with the gonadal* sex, and the external genitalia may be ambiguous. Female pseudo-hermaphrodites have a normal female chromosome* pattern (46 XX) and normal ovarian tissue, but varying degrees of masculinization of their external genitalia such as clitoral* enlargement and fusion of the labia*; however, the uterus and tubes are present as well as the ovaries and reproductive function is therefore possible after treatment. The condition may be the result of adrenal* cortical hyperplasia or occur in a female fetus after maternal ingestion in pregnancy of progestogens* with androgenic* effects (as present in some oral contraceptives).

Male pseudo-hermaphrodites have normal testes (often undescended*) and the normal male chromosome pattern (46 XY), but female bodily features; this results from a lack of androgen receptors in the genital tissues. In the testicular* feminization syndrome, the individual has a 46 XY karyotype* and produces testosterone* which is inactive due to absence of androgen receptors in the developing reproductive system. There is a vagina which ends as a blind pouch. The cervix, uterus, tubes and ovaries are absent. There is marked breast enlargement at puberty* and little pubic or axillary hair growth. The testes remain in the pelvis or inguinal canal with an increased risk of malignancy. Their removal is recommended for this reason.

herpes: a large group of viruses*. Human herpes simplex, type I, affects mainly the oral cavity with shallow painful ulcers of the lips and mouth (cold sores). Herpes simplex type 2 is usually sexually* transmitted and produces painful ulcers of the penis* or vulva*, vagina* and cervix* (see genital herpes). Outbreaks respond to treatment with local or systemic anti-viral drugs but the disease is often recurrent due to reactivation of virus that can remain latent in nerve cells. Other herpes viruses include herpes zoster (which causes chickenpox* and shingles), cytomegalovirus* and Epstein–Barr virus (which causes glandular fever).

heterotopic pregnancy: the simultaneous presence of an intra-uterine and an extra-uterine*, usually tubal, pregnancy. This condition is rare in normal conceptions, but found somewhat more frequently following IVF* and embryo* transfer.

heterozygote: an individual in whom the maternal and paternal versions (alleles*) of a gene* are different. For example, someone who is a heterozygote with respect to the cystic fibrosis gene has, in each of their cells, one healthy version of the cystic fibrosis gene and one faulty version. Such an individual is said to be heterozygous for the gene in question. (See homozygote.)

hirsutism: excessive amounts of facial or bodily hair in otherwise normally feminine women. In many cases there is a racial or familial element, but there may be an underlying hormonal* abnormality. Of these, the commonest is polycystic* ovarian syndrome; adrenal hyperplasia* and masculinizing ovarian tumours are other causes.

homozygote: an individual in whom the maternal and paternal versions (alleles*) of a gene* are the same. For example, someone who has two healthy versions of the cystic fibrosis gene is said to be a homozygote, but so too is someone both of whose versions of the cystic fibrosis gene are faulty. (See heterozygote.)

hormone: a chemical substance secreted by a ductless (endocrine*) gland into the blood stream and which exerts its action on distant, specific target cells or organs. Examples include thyroxine, secreted by the thyroid* gland, oestrogen* from the ovaries* and testosterone* from the testes*.

hormone assay: see assay.

hormone replacement therapy (HRT): the administration of ovarian hormones (usually both oestrogens* and progestogens*) to women after the menopause*, or after bilateral oophorectomy*, in order to relieve menopausal symptoms and prevent postmenopausal changes such as osteoporosis*. Administration can be in the form of tablets, injections, implants or skin patches.

In ART*, hormone replacement therapy may be used after suppression of endogenous hormones so that endometrial* development can be regulated; this is done to regularise irregular cycles or to synchronize two women's cycles for egg* donation.

Men with testosterone* deficiency due to anorchism* or Klinefelter's* syndrome require HRT with testosterone injections or implants.

Huehner's test: see post-coital test.

human chorionic gonadotrophin (hCG): this gonadotrophin* is produced by the trophectoderm* and, after implantation* has occurred, by the placenta*. It stimulates the corpus* luteum to continue producing oestradiol* and progesterone* and thus defer menstruation*. Pregnancy* tests specifically detect the β chain in blood or urine. The concentration of hCG doubles each day in early pregnancy if the pregnancy is developing normally. Lower concentrations may suggest an extra-uterine* pregnancy. hCG concentrations are greatly increased in patients with a hydatidiform* mole or choriocarcinoma*.

Because of the structural similarity with LH*, hCG is used to simulate the LH* surge during ovulation* induction. It may also be used to support the luteal* phase of cycles when GnRH* analogues have been administered.

In males, hCG has the same action on the Leydig* cells as LH*. It is used to treat hypogonadotrophic* hypogonadism and delayed male puberty* when stimulation of the Leydig* cells results in increased androgen* secretion.

Human Fertilisation and Embryology Act: the act passed in 1990 by the UK Parliament to control procedures employed in assisted* reproduction techniques in the UK.

The Act legislates on the handling and storage of embryos* created *in vitro* and of donated gametes*; it stipulates conditions under which research on human embryos* may be performed and also legislates on the legal status and registration of children born as a result of gamete or embryo donation. The Act also contains minor amendments to the 1967 Abortion Act and the 1985 Surrogacy Act.

The Act established the Human* Fertilisation and Embryology Authority (HFEA) to enforce the legislation and, among its many other functions, to license and inspect clinics in which embryos or donated gametes are handled or stored and to ensure the maintenance of patient confidentiality*. Severe penalties (suspension of clinic, fines, imprisonment) are prescribed for offences against the Act.

Human Fertilisation and Embryology Authority (HFEA): this body was set up in 1991 by Act of Parliament (1990) to regulate all procedures which involve the handling or storage of embryos* or donated gametes*, or the conduct of research on human embryos in the UK.

The Authority inspects and licenses clinics in which such procedures are carried out, prescribes necessary qualifications for personnel working in such clinics and ensures high standards of practice. It recommends the provision of opportunities for counselling* in clinics and issues guidelines relating to clinic practice, social and ethical* issues, confidentiality* and research.

Apart from emphasizing the clinics' obligations to patients and donors, the Authority stresses that its overriding consideration is the welfare of the child(ren) to be born. The Authority, which has replaced the earlier Voluntary* Licensing Authority and the Interim* Licensing Authority, publishes annual reports on its work which also summarise the results of treatments at the licensed centres and list new developments in infertility treatment, details of licensed centres and current research projects.

human immunodeficiency virus (HIV):

this virus* causes AIDS* and may be transmitted by sexual activity (both heterosexual and male to male homosexual), by transfer of body fluids (blood, semen, vaginal secretion, breast milk) or vertically, from mother to fetus during pregnancy and/or delivery. Transmission in a healthcare setting is rare but has occurred as a result of needlestick injuries, transfusion of infected blood or blood products, donor* insemination and transplantation of infected organs.

Since most HIV-infected individuals are symptom-free for many years after acquiring the infection, the diagnosis is made by detecting antibodies* to the virus* in the patient's blood. Antibody production takes up to three months after the infection is acquired (the 'window period') during which time an individual may be infected and potentially infectious but negative on antibody testing. In many assisted reproduction clinics, all patients are tested for HIV. Prior to any form of tissue donation, HIV testing of the donor is required. In the case of semen*

donation, the specimen is frozen and only released for use when, after a quarantine period of at least three (usually six) months, the donor has been retested and shown still to be negative.

Donated oocytes and embryos may also be quarantined, but freezing results in lower success rates. In view of the low risk of HIV among oocyte donors, some clinics use donated oocytes without freezing quarantine. In all assisted reproduction units, strict controls are in place to prevent infection or contamination of all specimens.

Providing assisted reproduction services for couples where one or both members are HIV-infected is controversial because of the limited life expectancy of the sufferer, the risk of transmission to the fetus if it is the mother who is HIV-positive and potential risks to clinic staff during the procedures involved.

human menopausal gonadotrophin (hMG):

see gonadotrophins. HMG preparations are used for ovarian* stimulation and multiple follicular* development. Proprietory brands include Humegon, Metrodin, Normegon, Orgafol and Pergonal. In men, hMG is used to treat hypogonadotrophic* hypogonadism.

human papilloma virus (HPV):

there are more than 70 different subtypes of this virus*, identified by differences in their genetic structure and responsible for several human diseases including common warts, verrucae and genital warts*. HPV infection is extremely common and the virus is carried by the majority of individuals without producing disease.

The development of clinical warts in individuals infected with genital subtypes HPV 6 and 11 may be precipitated by local factors such as trauma or reduced immunity in pregnancy. Some HPV types are involved in the development of CIN* and cervical cancer; however, co-factors are also involved and among those infected with an oncogenic* (cancer-producing) type such as HPV 16 only a small proportion of individuals will develop clinical disease. Cervical HPV infection is diagnosed by biopsy* or cytology*; treatment is only indicated if there is co-existing CIN as spontaneous clearance may occur. HPV may also play a role in the development of pre-malignant or malignant lesions in the vulva*.

Huntingdon's chorea: a rare neurological condition characterized by the degeneration of the nervous system. Affected people find motor co-ordination difficult so that their hands shake and they have problems with balance. As the condition worsens they find it more and more difficult to look after themselves. The disease usually manifests itself in people aged between 30 and 50, and death generally follows within five to ten years. The condition is caused by the possession of a mutant autosomal* dominant* allele*. This means that individuals homozygous* or heterozygous* for the allele are affected. In Britain the average incidence of people with the mutant allele is about 7 per 100 000. However, in some places, notably in the Moray Firth area in Scotland, the condition is almost one hundred times more frequent.

hyaluronidase: an enzyme* capable of digesting hyaluronic acid. Hyaluronic acid is a component of the mucus surrounding the expanded cumulus* oophorus. Hyaluronidase is contained in the acrosome* of spermatozoa, ready to disperse the cumulus and enable fertilization* to take place. Hyaluronidase may be used in embryology to remove cumulus cells before micromanipulation* of the oocyte.

hydatidiform mole: an abnormality of the placenta* in which the chorionic villi (see chorion) become swollen and distended with fluid as a result of neoplastic changes. The placenta thus comes to resemble a bunch of grapes with many hundreds of vesicles varying in size from a pin head to a cherry. Usually there is no fetus, but rarely one is found in a partial mole.

Bleeding occurs late in the first or early in the second trimester*. The condition is diagnosed by ultrasound scanning* and abnormally high concentrations of hCG* in blood or urine. As the pregnancy is non-viable and there is a high risk of haemorrhage, treatment is by evacuation of the uterus.

The incidence in Western women is about one in 2000, but it is much higher in women living around the Pacific rim. A small number of moles progress to a choriocarcinoma* which will continue to secrete hCG*. For this reason, after treatment for hydatidiform mole, prolonged follow-up by measuring serum hCG concentrations is essential. Some moles are associated with triploidy* with one maternal and two paternal sets of chromosomes*; others are believed to be the result of fertilization* of an oocyte with a degenerated nucleus* by a duplicated haploid* spermatozoon.

Hydramnios: an excessive amount of amniotic fluid (see amniotic cavity): usually this is accepted as meaning more than 2 litres, but as measurement is difficult, the clinical definition is an excess of fluid sufficient to cause problems in pregnancy or labour. The condition is more common in women with diabetes* or multiple* pregnancies, and is particularly associated with certain fetal abnormalities such as tracheo-oesophageal fistula, duodenal atresia and neural* tube defects. For the mother there is marked discomfort, and a higher incidence of pre-eclampsia* and placental separation. The risks to the fetus* are considerable and include prematurity*, malpresentation, placental separation, prolapse of the umbilical* cord and congenital* malformations.

hydrocele: a primary hydrocele is a tense, painless collection of fluid of unknown origin around the testicle*. The fluid is restricted to the tunica* vaginalis. A secondary hydrocele is less tense with less fluid and can occur after epididymitis*, orchitis* or in association with a testicular tumour. A hydrocele of the cord is an encysted fluid collection of the spermatic* cord due to incomplete obliteration of the processus vaginalis. Hydroceles do not contain spermatozoa and do not cause male infertility.

hydrosalpinx (Fig. 13b): fluid distension of the Fallopian* tube when the abdominal* ostium has become occluded. This usually follows a tubal infection. Hydrosalpinx is the commonest form of tubal occlusion. The condition is diagnosed by hysterosalpingography* and laparoscopy* when particular attention is paid to the size of the hydrosalpinx, the thickness of the walls and the extent of surrounding adhesions*.

Favourable cases are treated by tubal microsurgery*. If this fails or if the condition is too severe to attempt surgery the patient should be offered treatment by IVF*. Success rates for IVF* are thought to be lower in patients with hydrosalpinx compared with those infertile due to other causes, possibly due to periodic drainage of tubal fluid into the uterine* cavity.

hymen (Fig. 27): a thin membrane, covered on both sides by mucosa, which stretches across the entrance to the vagina*. The hymen varies considerably in thickness. If totally imperforate, menstrual blood cannot escape and haematocolpos* results. A tough inelastic hymen can prevent adequate coitus* and is occasionally found in the course of infertility investigations.

hyperactivation: a type of erratic activity of spermatozoa* which occurs after capacitation* and can be used as an indicator of the sperms' ability to fertilize.

hyperandrogenism: changes caused by abnormally high androgen* concentrations in women. The milder forms include hirsutism* and acne and are often associated with polycystic* ovarian syndrome. The more severe forms include baldness, deepening of the voice, loss of breast tissue and hypertrophy of the clitoris and are found in association with the rare masculinizing tumours of the ovary or in adrenal* hyperplasia.

hypergonadotrophic hypogonadism: see hypogonadism.

hyperplasia: overgrowth of a tissue due to excessive cell proliferation.

hyperprolactinaemia: raised concentrations of the hormone prolactin* in the blood. The symptoms of galactorrhoea*, amenorrhoea* and infertility are only seen if the blood concentration of prolactin* is above 2500 iu/L. Lower concentrations are associated with acute stress and polycystic* ovarian syndrome and are usually asymptomatic.

The condition is caused by certain drugs (narcotics, tranquillizers, antidepressants and others), by a benign adenoma* of the pituitary* gland or by thyroid* deficiency. Pituitary adenomas (prolactinoma) account for over 30% of all cases: they may be minute in size (micro-adenoma) and can only be diagnosed by X-rays and especially CT and MRI scans. Treatment is either medical with long term dopamine* antagonists such as bromocriptine* or surgical, and the prospects for fertility are good following treatment.

Occasionally hyperprolactinaemia occurs in men, when it usually presents with impotence*, but only rarely with infertility.

hyperstimulation: excessive response of the ovaries to ovarian* stimulation. See ovarian hyperstimulation syndrome (OHSS).

hypertension: raised blood* pressure, usually defined as a systolic blood pressure greater than 140 mmHg and/or a diastolic greater than 90 mmHg. In most cases the cause of hypertension is unknown, but it may be secondary to kidney disease, certain endocrine* disorders and pre-eclampsia*. The incidence increases with age. It is usually discovered by routine blood pressure measurement and there may be no symptoms. Headache is the commonest presenting symptom, but the first sign may be a stroke or heart failure. Pregnant women with hypertension need particularly good antenatal care as there are risks of exacerbation as well as the development of pre-eclampsia* in pregnancy.

hyperthecosis: also known as sclerocystic disease of the ovaries: hyperplasia* of the theca* cells with marked ovarian enlargement and dysfunction resulting in hirsutism*, obesity*, menstrual* irregularities and infertility*. This is a histological diagnosis and probably represents a late stage of the Stein*–Leventhal and polycystic* ovarian syndromes.

hyperthyroidism: over activity of the thyroid* gland with increasing amounts of thyroid hormone in the blood stream. This condition is also known as thyrotoxicosis and, when associated with eye changes, Graves' disease. A goitre is frequently present.

Symptoms include increased appetite, loss of weight, palpitations, tremor, heat intolerance and perspiration. In women, menstrual disturbances are frequent, with amenorrhoea*, oligomenorrhoea* and anovulation* the commonest. Fertility is frequently reduced, but becomes normal following treatment of the thyroid condition. However, pregnancy can occur in untreated women suffering from thyrotoxicosis. In men, hyperthyroidism can cause gynaecomastia* and infertility.

hypogonadism: failure of the gonads* (testes* or ovaries*) to produce sex hormones or gametes*, or both. Secondary sexual* characteristics are absent or regress.

The clinical features depend on whether the onset of gonadal failure is before or after puberty*. If pre-pubertal, both sexes exhibit general bodily immaturity, minimal pubic and axillary hair growth, and greater height than average because the growth plates (epiphyses) of long bones fail to close due to lack of oestradiol* or testosterone*. Girls have primary amenorrhoea* and no breast development. Boys have small testes, no voice changes and no facial hair growth.

If hypogonadism occurs after puberty, there is regression of secondary sexual characteristics and infertility. Women have secondary amenorrhoea, breast regression, vaginal dryness and other symptoms of oestrogen withdrawal (see premature ovarian failure). Men develop azoospermia* or severe oligospermia* and have less facial hair growth and possibly diminished libido.

Primary hygonadism, due to ovarian* or testicular* failure, is associated with raised gonadotrophin* (FSH* and LH*) and low oestradiol and testosterone concentrations (hypergonadotrophic hypogonadism). In women, the condition may be congenital (e.g. Turner's* syndrome and other forms of ovarian agenesis) or acquired (bilateral oophorectomy*, irradiation, chemotherapy).

In men, congenital causes include Klinefelter's* syndrome, Sertoli*-cell-only syndrome and undescended* testes, whilst acquired causes include mumps* orchitis*, orchidectomy*, irradiation and chemotherapy.

There is no known treatment which will initiate oogenesis* or spermatogenesis* in patients with primary gonadal failure. Treatment with gonadotrophins or GnRH* analogues is inappropriate. Women will require treatment with hormone* replacement therapy (HRT), and egg* donation if pregnancy is desired. Recent results in men reveal that 50% of those with primary testicular failure have areas of normal spermatogenesis from which spermatozoa can be retrieved by TESE* for ICSI*. In these patients, HRT should be withheld until fertility treatment is completed, in order to avoid pituitary suppression.

Secondary hypogonadism is due to pituitary* or hypothalamic* disturbances: see hypogonadotrophic hypogonadism.

hypogonadotrophic hypogonadism: this form of hypogonadism* results from failure of normal pituitary function or failure by the hypothalamus* to produce GnRH*. Consequently gonadotrophin* (FSH* & LH*) and oestradiol*/testosterone* concentrations are low.

In women, the hypogonadism may result from conditions such as Sheehan's* syndrome, pituitary* tumours, or be related to nutritional disturbances (anorexia* nervosa) or excessively strenuous athletic activities. The uterus and ovaries are small, there is amenorrhoea* and a risk of osteoporosis*; there is no reponse to treatment with clomiphene citrate*. These patients respond well to treatment with hMG* or pulsatile GnRH.

The condition is rare in men and is either congenital (see Kallmann's syndrome), or due to head injury or to disease or tumour of the pituitary* gland. Men affected before puberty, unless treatment of the testosterone* deficiency is started before puberty*, have a eunuchoidal appearance with scanty body hair, gynaecomastia*, low muscle mass and unbroken voice. They have small testes*, are azoospermic* and, sometimes, impotent*. Replacement therapy with hCG* and hMG* or pulsatile GnRH* is usually effective in stimulating sperm production, although this may take over a year.

hypomenorrhoea: regular menstrual bleeding with a reduction in both duration and amount of flow. Usually this is a constitutional variation from the normal and of little significance with no reduction in fertility. If there is infertility, hormone levels should be checked, and a hysteroscopy* performed to exclude intra-uterine adhesions (see Asherman's syndrome).

hypo-osmotic swelling test: a diagnostic test for the viability of spermatozoa*. Spermatozoa are placed in diluted saline: if their tails swell, they are alive.

hypopituitarism: failure of the anterior lobe of the pituitary* gland to produce adequate amounts of pituitary hormones. If this affects only the FSH* and LH* output, hypogonadotrophic* hypogonadism will result. Other hormone* deficiencies may occur as a result of failure of growth hormone*, thyroid* stimulating or adrenal* corticotrophic hormone production. In some cases of hypopituitarism, the cause is a tumour of the pituitary gland or surrounding tissues; rarely in women the cause is a postpartum necrosis associated with excessive blood loss and shock in the third stage of labour (see Sheehan's syndrome).

hypospadias: a congenital abnormality of the penis* in which urine is passed through an abnormally placed opening on the undersurface of the body of the penis. This condition is normally treated by plastic reconstructive surgery in childhood. Unless there is an associated abnormality of the testes* or male genital tract, fertility is normal. Sometimes, unsuccessful repair may interfere with ejaculation* or sperm deposition in the upper vagina. Treatment then is by artificial* insemination with the partner's semen (AIH).

hypothalamus (Fig. 12): part of the forebrain with nervous connections to the thalamus and other parts of the

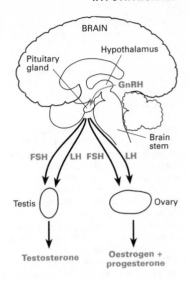

Fig. **12**. The Hypothalamic – Pituitary – Gonadal Axis.

brain. It is involved in the control of certain autonomic functions such as body temperature, sleep, thirst, appetite and fluid balance.

Anatomically, the hypothalamus is closely linked to the pituitary* gland with which it communicates by both nerve pathways and a specialized blood circulation, the hypothalamic–portal venous system. Through the release of gonadotrophin* releasing hormone (GnRH), the hypothalamus regulates the pituitary output of FSH* and LH* which in turn act on the ovaries to control the ovarian and menstrual* cycles, and on the testes to promote the secretion of androgens* and spermatogenesis*.

hypothyroidism: subnormal activity of the thyroid* gland resulting in reduced output of thyroid hormone. In childhood this may lead to cretinism and in adults to myxoedema*. A goitre is frequently present. In women hypothyroidism often causes menstrual disorders (prolonged, irregular or heavy periods, or amenorrhoea*) and anovulation*. Galactorrhoea* may occur. Fertility is greatly reduced, and if pregnancy does occur, there is a risk of miscarriage* or stillbirth*. Treatment with thyroxine restores normal fertility.

In men hypothyroidism can cause impotence* and may interfere with spermatogenesis*.

hyskon: a highly viscous solution of dextran in dextrose, used as a fluid medium to dilate the uterine* cavity at hysteroscopy*.

hysterectomy: the surgical operation to excise the uterus*. This can be done abdominally or vaginally. The abdominal operation is called total hysterectomy if the cervix* is removed as well as the body of the uterus and subtotal if the cervix is retained. The Fallopian* tubes and ovaries* may also be removed (especially in postmenopausal women) and the operation is then named total hysterectomy and bilateral salpingo-oophorectomy. Recently laparoscopic assisted techniques have been developed for hysterectomy whilst the develpment of endometrial* ablation in suitable cases may avoid hysterectomy.

Indications for the operation include menorrhagia*, severe endometriosis*, benign (fibroids*) or malignant tumours of the uterus or cervix. In premenopausal women who have had a hysterectomy, ovarian* failure may develop earlier than the normal menopause*. Young women who have had a hysterectomy with preservation of at least one ovary, may be assisted to have children by surrogacy*, using their own oocytes* and their partners' spermatozoa for IVF* and embryo transfer into the surrogate.

hystero-salpingography (Figs. 13a+b): radiological visualization of the uterine* cavity and the lumen of the Fallopian* tubes: a radio-opaque solution (water soluble is preferred to oil soluble) is injected via a special cannula through the cervical* canal and X-ray pictures are taken, giving an outline of the uterus and tubes. The primary purpose is to demonstrate tubal patency or occlusion but other tubal abnormalities such as rigidity due to scarring, irregularity of the lumen, loss of mucosal folds, and cornual polyps can also be identified. Uterine abnormalities may be revealed, such as the presence of polyps*, submucous fibroids*, intra-uterine adhesions*, enlargement and distortion of the cavity due to intra mural fibroids* or congenital malformations. This investigation is complementary to laparoscopy* which provides a view of the external appearance of the uterus and Fallopian* tubes, and the pelvis as a whole.

hysteroscopy: direct visualization of the uterine* cavity via a narrow endoscope* inserted through the cervix*. For the examination, the uterine cavity is distended by Hyskon*, saline or carbon dioxide. Originally, hysteroscopy was designed for the diagnosis of conditions such as uterine polyps*, submucous fibroids*, intra-uterine adhesions*, uterine septa, malignancy and the presence of retained* products of conception or retained intra-uterine* contraceptive devices. It is now also

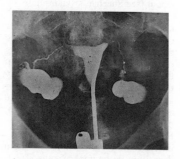

Fig. 13. Hysterosalpingography (HSG).

13.a. Normal HSG: the injected contrast medium outlines the uterine cavity and the thin, elongated, graceful Fallopian tubes. There is a little spill of contrast medium into the peritoneal cavity on the left and more on the right side where the contrast medium is coated over the surface of a loop of bowel.

13.b. HSG showing bilateral hydrosalpinges. The proximal interstitial and isthmic portions of the tubes are normal, but the ampullae are grossly dilated and there is no spill from the abdominal ostia into the peritoneal cavity.

employed in the treatment of uterine septa or intra-uterine adhesions*, removal of submucous fibroids*, and for endometrial ablation. It is also used to visualize the cornual openings of the Fallopian* tubes and to cannulate them (see falloposcopy).

hysterotomy: incision into the wall of the uterus to gain access to the cavity. This used to be done in the course of removing submucous fibroids or uterine septa, but these are now treated via the hysteroscope*. The term is usually employed to describe a miniature Caesarean section for termination of a pregnancy which is too advanced for removal by the vaginal route or for the evacuation of a hydatidiform* mole, but even for these indications hysterotomy is now rarely required.

I

iatrogenic infertility: infertility caused by a medical or surgical event. For example, pelvic infections can be caused by curettage*, termination of pregnancy, hysterosalpingography* or insertion of an IUCD* and can lead to tubal damage or adhesion* formation. Adhesions, interfering with the tubal ovum* pick-up mechanism, can also be caused by surgical operations such as ovarian cystectomy or myomectomy*. Intra-uterine adhesions (see Asherman's* syndrome) can be caused by curettage following miscarriage or delivery. Some operations on the cervix can destroy the columnar epithelium of the cervical canal and cause a deficiency of cervical mucus*.

In men, injury to the vas* deferens can occur during hernia repair or varicocele* ligation and to the epididymis* during hydrocele* repair.

Sterilization operations are obvious causes of iatrogenic infertility in both sexes and the use of chemotherapy or radiotherapy may cause temporary or permanent damage to the gonads*.

ICSI: see intra-cytoplasmic sperm injection.

identical twins: see multiple pregnancy.

idiopathic infertility: see unexplained infertility.

immotile cilia syndrome: an autosomal* recessive* disorder present in 1 in 20 000 men. The spermatozoa* are either all immotile or their motility is severely impaired due to structural abnormalities of the tail. The condition can be identified by electron microscopy and may affect ciliated* cells throughout the body. In half the cases it is associated with Kartagener's* syndrome.The infertility is managed by ICSI* using ejaculated spermatozoa, provided their viability has been confirmed by some movement or a positive hypo-osmotic* swelling test.

immunity: a state in which an individual is protected against subsequent disease by the presence of circulating antibodies*. This normally follows a successful immune response. Immunity can result from vaccination and/or exposure to the pathological agent. Immunity is normally measured using antibody* levels, but this is an imperfect measure of protection as individuals with antibodies can be reinfected.

immunoglobulin: see antibody.

immunobead test: a test to detect the presence of antisperm* antibodies. Immunobeads are microscopic polyacrylamide beads with anti-human immunoglobulin (Ig) antibodies* bound to their surface. They will attach to spermatozoa* which have such antibodies on their surface.

Two separate types of immunobeads, IgG and IgA, are used in the investigation of infertility. The direct immunobead test identifies antibodies attached to the surface of spermatozoa and is similar to the MAR* test. The indirect test identifies antisperm antibodies in the blood or seminal* plasma. IgG antibodies often appear following vasectomy* but may not interfere with sperm function. IgA antibodies are considered to be more significant in the identification of immunological* infertility; they occur in about 5% of infertile men, either naturally or in association with genito-urinary infection and are also found in 1% of infertile women. (See antisperm antibodies.)

immunological infertility: in women the cervical* mucus can contain antibodies* against spermatozoa*, causing immunological infertility. The postcoital* test (PCT) may show absent or reduced sperm motility, a 'shaking' phenomenon and/or agglutination* of the spermatozoa. Some authorities claim that 10 to 15% of women with unexplained* infertility have sperm immobilizing antibodies in the serum or cervical mucus, but others point out that such antibodies can also be detected in fertile women. Probably the significance of the antibodies is in proportion to their titre.

In men, antisperm* antibodies are the result of an auto-immune* response to surgical interference, trauma or infection and are thought to be responsible for up to 10% of unexplained* male infertility. Treatment of immunological infertility can be with corticosteroids to suppress the immune response (see cortisone), but there is a risk of severe side effects. IVF* is very effective. (See also antisperm antibodies, immunobead test.)

implantation: the process by which the blastocyst* becomes embedded in the decidual* lining of the uterus* at the beginning of pregnancy. In humans, implantation comprises apposition, when the blastocyst becomes closely apposed to the decidua*, adhesion when it first attaches to the decidua (see adhesion molecules), and penetration when it reaches the basement membrane and stroma of the uterus and establishes contact with the maternal circulation. Implantation occurs about 7 days after ovulation*. For it to be successful, the blastocyst must escape from the zona* pellucida (see hatching), develop trophoblastic* microvilli and send signals by hCG* secretion to the mother. Meanwhile the endometrium*, under the influence of progesterone*, has thickened, become more vascular and is transformed into the decidua*.

impotence: the inability of the penis* to develop or maintain an erection* adequate for intercourse. This is also known as erectile impotence or erectile dysfunction and differs from ejaculatory* impotence. Men with erectile impotence can reach orgasm* and ejaculate in response to penile stimulation whilst men with ejaculatory impotence may have normal erection but cannot reach orgasm or ejaculate despite penile stimulation.

The causes and mechanism of both types of impotence are often the same and include marital or psychological problems, diabetes*, Peyronie's* disease (fibrosis of the penis), disturbances of blood flow and side effects of drugs, especially anti-hypertensives and anti-depressants. Less common causes are pituitary* tumours (including prolactin* secreting microadenomas), testosterone* insufficiency due to hypogonadism*, spinal* injury and neurological conditions affecting the autonomic nervous system.

In the treatment of infertility, impotence, whether erectile or ejaculatory, can be regarded as a purely mechanical problem, preventing the transmission of spermatozoa from male to female; sperm production and function are usually normal and treatment with artificial* insemination (AIH) is commonly successful. (See also ejaculatory failure, retrograde ejaculation, artificial insemination.)

imprinting: a term used in two senses. (1) A form of learning in which an animal, early in its development, passes through a brief sensitive period during which it learns to recognize certain stimuli and subsequently respond to them in a characteristic fashion. For example, ducklings in the first couple of days after they hatch learn to follow their mother. If presented, experimentally, with a moving box or other object instead of their mother, they 'learn' that this is their mother and subsequently follow it faithfully. In humans, such imprinting, though still significant, is probably less important than in other mammals and birds. (2) Genomic imprinting is a phenomenon which results in the maternal and paternal chromosomes* contributing differently to early development.

infertility: failure to conceive after regular unprotected intercourse: 70% of couples will achieve a pregnancy by the end of one year and 85% after two years. Failure to conceive after one year is generally regarded as an indication to start investigations and treatment, but in couples where the woman is 35 years or over (see age) investigations should be started earlier. Epidemiological surveys show that about 1 in 6 couples have an infertility problem at some time in their lives. Infertility is primary when a pregnancy has never been achieved, or secondary when there is no further conception following one or more previous pregnancies or miscarriages.

The chief causes of female infertility are failure of ovulation*, disease of the Fallopian* tubes, cervical* mucus defects or pelvic factors such as fibroids* and endometriosis* which are associated with infertility in some cases. In the male, the semen* analysis may be abnormal due to deficiencies in sperm number, motility, morphology or fertilizing ability (see sperm* dysfunction) or the spermatozoa* may be coated with antisperm* antibodies. Coital* factors include infrequent or incorrectly timed* intercourse; other factors such as vaginimus*, impotence*, ejaculatory* dysfunction or dyspareunia*, if not revealed in the history, can be detected by a negative post-coital* test. In some couples no definite cause of infertility is found and treatment is empirical (see unexplained infertility).

The management of infertility entails detailed history taking from both partners (including their fertility with previous partners), followed by physical examination. Routine investigations include semen* analysis, a postcoital* test, tests of ovulation* (such as basal* body temperature, mid-luteal* serum progesterone measurement, ultrasound* ovarian scans and endometrial biopsy*) and investigation of the Fallopian* tubes and pelvic structures by hysterosalpingography*, laparoscopy* and possibly fallopos-copy* and salpingoscopy*. Only by following such steps can a proper diagnosis be made and rational treatment given.

inflammation: the cellular* response to a noxious stimulus, such as bacterial* or viral* infection, trauma, chemical or thermal injury. Acute inflammatory conditions in the genital tracts can cause infertility in both men and women: acute salpingitis* will interfere with fertilization* and sperm* or oocyte* transport; endometritis* prevents implantation*; vaginal or cervical infections may interfere with sperm survival. In the male, epididym-itis* and orchitis* depress spermatogenesis*.

Chronic inflammatory conditions may follow episodes of acute or in-adequately treated inflammation; the resultant scarring can cause mechanical infertility due to obstruction or blockage of the Fallopian* tubes, the epididymis* or the vas* deferens. In women the likelihood of permanent tubal damage is directly related to the number of episodes of salpingitis experienced.

infundibulum (Figs. 8, 26): the dilated, trumpet-shaped portion of the Fallopian* tube which is its opening into the abdominal cavity. The fimbriae* project from the rim of the infundibulum and have an important role in the ovum* pick-up mechanism. (See abdominal ostium, Fallopian tube, fimbriae.)

inhibin: a hormone*, existing in various forms, produced by the ovaries* and testes*. In women, inhibin B is produced by the dominant follicle* and results in suppression of FSH* concentrations and thus atresia* of the other developing follicles. Inhibin A is produced by both the follicle and the corpus* luteum, but its role is unclear. Inhibin A has recently been included in the quadruple test as an antenatal marker for Down's* syndrome.

In men, inhibin is produced by the testis in response to spermatogenesis*, which, by negative feedback to the hypothalamus* and pituitary* gland, limits the secretion of FSH*.

inner cell mass: the cells of the blastocyst* which form the body of the embryo.

insemination: see artificial insemination; also intra-peritoneal, intra-uterine and subzonal insemination.

in situ hybridization: see fluorescence *in situ* hybridization.

insufflation: see tubal insufflation.

intercourse: see coitus, timed intercourse.

Interim Licensing Authority: title adopted by the Voluntary* Licensing Authority (VLA) from 1989 until the setting up of the Human* Fertilisation and Embryology Authority (HFEA) in 1991.

internal cervical os (Fig. 26): the opening of the upper end of the cervical canal into the uterine cavity. (See cervix, cervical incompetence.)

intersex: the condition in which there are varying degrees of masculinization of the female or feminization of the male. The sexual organs are ambiguous at birth so that assignment of gender* poses difficulty. Examples are female babies whose enlarged clitoris* at birth (due to hormonal stimulation in the adrenogenital* syndrome) is mistaken for a penis*, or males in whom a small penis with hypospadias*, bifid (split) scrotum* and failure of testicular descent leads to a false diagnosis of being female.

In other cases, the genital organs do not correspond with the genetic sex: for example in XY 'females', due to androgen* sensitivity, intra-uterine testicular failure or errors in testosterone* biosynthesis. Most of these patients have a short vagina, absent uterus and abnormally positioned gonads*. Such gonads have an increased risk of malignancy and should be removed. (See also hermaphroditism.)

interstitial cells: see Leydig cells, testis.

interstitial pregnancy (*syn.* cornual pregnancy): pregnancy occurring in that part of the Fallopian* tube which passes through the uterine musculature. This is an uncommon type of extrauterine* pregnancy and can present difficulties in diagnosis and management.

intra-cytoplasmic sperm injection (ICSI): (Fig. 1.4): the injection of a single spermatozoon* into the cytoplasm* of the oocyte*. This recently developed technique has changed and greatly improved the management of male infertility due to severe oligozoospermia*. Before the introduction of ICSI, traditional IVF* required more than about half a million progressively motile spermatozoa for a good chance of fertilization*: ICSI requires only one spermatozoon to be injected into each oocyte. Sperm* dysfunction may also be overcome by ICSI since more than 50% of oocytes usually fertilize normally, regardless of the quality of the sperm injected, provided it is viable.

Since so few spermatozoa are required, the indications for ICSI have been expanded to include nearly all men with serious infertility. Ejaculates* of the poorest quality, as well as acrosome*-less spermatozoa (see globozoospermia), immature epididymal and testicular spermatozoa

and round spermatids* (maturation arrest) have been used to generate embryos. About one third of men with azoospermia*, even those with atrophic*, small testes* and grossly elevated FSH* levels, have some areas of normal sperm production in the testes which can be aspirated (TESA*) or biopsied* to collect spermatozoa for ICSI. ICSI has also led to minimally invasive methods of surgical sperm retrieval in obstructive* azoospermia which can be carried out under local anaesthesia. Donor* insemination (DI) is thus employed less frequently in the modern management of male infertility.

Careful monitoring of ICSI generated embryos and children born has to date shown no significant increase in fetal abnormalities, although an apparent increase in sex chromosome anomalies remains to be confirmed. However, testicular failure causing azoospermia and severe oligozoospermia is associated with an abnormal karyotype* in 10 to 15% of cases and ICSI circumvents the natural events of sperm selection and maturation, so the genetic evaluation of the male partner has become essential as a precaution against the transmission of mutations*.

intra-peritoneal insemination: also known as direct intra-peritoneal insemination or DIPI: an assisted* reproduction technique in which prepared* specimens of spermatozoa* are injected into the peritoneal cavity, through the posterior vaginal fornix*, at the time of ovulation*. Ovarian* stimulation may or may not be used. The main indications for this technique are male factor infertility, immunological* infertility due to antisperm* antibodies or unexplained* infertility. The success rate of DIPI is variable and its value questionable. It is employed less, as intra-uterine* insemination and ICSI* are more widely used.

intra-tubal adhesions: adhesions* resulting from inflammation* of the endosalpinx*, usually following tubal infection or tubal pregnancy (see extrauterine pregnancy). Adhesions in the lumen of the Fallopian* tubes can cause infertility or tubal pregnancy. Visualization by falloposcopy* is now possible and their presence is a contraindication to tubal surgery in women suffering from tubal infertility: under such circumstances the results are better from treatment by IVF*.

intra-uterine contraceptive device (IUCD): a large variety of mechanical devices, inserted into the uterine* cavity via the cervical* canal, have been produced as a form of contraception*. The rings, coils, spirals and other shapes formerly made of gold, silver, stainless steel and other materials have now been replaced by plastic devices; some of these have copper thread (which is spermicidal) wound round the stem and others contain progestogens* which reduce menstrual loss and produce an impenetrable cervical* mucus and unresponsive endometrium*.

There is still disagreement about the mode of action, but interference with sperm migration through the uterus, possibly with fertilization* and with implantation* of the blastocyst* all operate. Most IUCDs have threads which protrude from the cervix* into the upper vagina. Their presence indicates that the IUCD is properly situated in the uterus and they also facilitate removal. Some forms of threads have been incriminated as a cause of ascending infection and threadless devices are now undergoing trial.

Complications of IUCDs include perforation of the uterus at insertion, spontaneous expulsion, heavy menstrual losses, dysmenorrhoea* and infection. Pregnancy rates are low, but if pregnancy should occur, there is a somewhat higher risk of extra-uterine* pregnancy in women using an IUCD. There is a slightly increased risk of pelvic infection (which could lead to infertility) in women who have never been pregnant and there is also evidence that in women who are at risk of sexually transmitted disease, IUCD use is associated with an increased incidence of pelvic infection. Nevertheless, in properly selected patients, this is a very efficient method of birth control.

Many gynaecologists will recommend IUCDs for spacing pregnancies or for contraception once the family is complete, but are reluctant to insert them for patients who have not yet proved their fertility. IUCDs are also used successfully for emergency contraception (see contraception) when inserted up to 5 days after unprotected intercourse.

intra-uterine insemination (IUI): an assisted* reproduction technique in which a prepared specimen of semen* (see sperm preparation) is injected by means of a cannula through the cervical* canal, directly into the uterine* cavity. The insemination is performed at the time of ovulation* as determined by ultrasound* or hormone* measurements, and is usually preceded by ovarian* stimulation. Previous investigations must have shown a normal uterus and normal Fallopian* tubes.

IUI is particularly useful in women with a deficient cervical* mucus. It is widely used for unexplained* infertility and mild endometriosis* before resorting to IVF*. Success in men with impaired sperm concentration or motility and those with antisperm* antibodies is doubtful. The technique is simpler and cheaper than IVF* and less objectionable to those who, on religious or personal grounds, may not wish to undergo IVF. Complications include ovarian* hyperstimulation, if stimulation is used, and multiple* pregnancy.

introitus: (*syn.* vestibule: Fig. 27): that part of the female lower genital tract which lies between the labia* minora and in front of the vaginal opening. The urethra* and ducts of Bartholin's* glands open into the introitus.

__in vitro__ **fertilization (IVF)**: the assisted* reproductive technology in which fertilization* is achieved in the laboratory (*lit.* in a glass dish—'*in vitro*'). Initially, IVF was used in women with irreparably damaged Fallopian* tubes, but as the technique has become more successful it is more widely used in conditions such as unexplained* infertility, severe endometriosis* and severe male infertility. More recent indications include pre-implantation* diagnosis, certain cases of premature* ovarian failure and egg* donation, and some cases of surrogacy*.

IVF consists of oocyte* collection just before ovulation*, which in most clinics is preceded by ovarian* stimulation so that more oocytes are available. The oocytes are mixed in specially prepared culture* media with a prepared specimen of semen* (see sperm preparation). Fertilization* and cleavage* are monitored by embryologists in the laboratory before transfer of one or more embryos at the 2 to 8 cells stage which is generally two to three days after oocyte collection. Embryo* transfer (ET) is performed through the cervical* canal with a special catheter. Luteal* phase support may be given, e.g. with progesterone*. A β hCG* pregnancy test is performed 14 days after embryo transfer and, if positive, an ultrasound* scan is performed two weeks later.

Only two or at the most three embryos are transferred in a treatment cycle in order to avoid high order multiple* pregnancies; spare embryos of good morphological appearance can be cryopreserved* for future use by the couple under treatment, or, with their consent, may be used for research. Oocyte collection and fertilization have reached a high degree of success, but the percentage of live-born* from a single treatment cycle is still disappointingly low at about 15% due to a high incidence of implantation* failure or very early miscarriage*. The chief complications of IVF occurring in women undergoing stimulation are ovarian* hyperstimulation (OHSS) and high order multiple* pregnancies. There is also a higher than average risk of extra-uterine* pregnancy.

The first pregnancy conceived by IVF was in fact a tubal pregnancy. The first live-birth following IVF was that of Louise Brown, on 25 July 1978, following pioneering treatment by Patrick Steptoe and Robert Edwards. IVF has been the most significant technique introduced into the management of infertility for decades and has led to the development of much new technology.

Such a procedure in which fertilization is achieved outside the body has raised serious ethical, legal, religious and political issues and debate on these continues. In the UK, IVF and other techniques which involve the handling of embryos or gametes* are controlled by the Human Fertilisation and Embryology Authority* (HFEA).

isthmus (Figs. 8 and 26): that part of the Fallopian* tube which extends from the outer angle of the uterus to the ampullary* portion of the tube. It is about 2.5 cm long, has a very narrow lumen (0.1 to 1 mm diameter), but thick muscular walls. The isthmus plays an important part in the transport of spermatozoa* and oocytes* and regulates the precise time of entry of the blastocyst* into the uterine cavity, about 80 hours after ovulation*.

Extra-uterine pregnancy* can ocur in the isthmus, though the ampulla* is a commoner site. When tubal pregnancy does occur in the isthmus, symptoms occur earlier due to the inability of the isthmus to expand, and perforation of the tube is more likely than tubal abortion.

isthmic occlusion: this is the second commonest site of tubal obstruction (hydrosalpinx*, occlusion at the abdominal ostium*, is the commonest). Occlusion in the isthmus* can be caused by utero–tubal infections, previous extra-uterine pregnancy*, tubal endometriosis* and polyps*. It is diagnosed by hysterosalpingography* and laparoscopy*. Treatment is by microsurgical* tubo-cornual anastomosis* or by IVF*. Some pregnancies have been achieved by falloposcopy*.

In present-day practice, the commonest cause of isthmic occlusion is a previous sterilization operation.

J

Johnsen score: a microscopic method of scoring the histological appearance of a testicular* biopsy*, based on the most advanced stage of spermatogenesis* present in each seminiferous* tube counted. A mean* score of 8 to 10 signifies normal spermatogenesis, below 8 impaired and below 2 no spermatogenesis.

K

Kallmann's syndrome: a rare congenital form of hypogonadotrophic* hypogonadism due to a single gene* defect associated with absence of hypothalamic GnRH* secretion. In males there is arrested puberty* in adolescents* and hypogonadism* in adults. The principal feature of the syndrome is anosmia* (loss of sense of smell), which is due to a midline brain development defect resulting in absence of the olfactory bulb (nerves of smell) and failure of migration of GnRH* producing neurons. This interferes with the development of the hypothalamic*–pituitary axis (Fig. 12) and access of GnRH to the pituitary* gland. There is also red–green colour blindness. Treatment with gonadotrophin* injections or a GnRH* pump usually improves testosterone* production and virilization, but the initiation of spermatogenesis* may be delayed with no spermatozoa in the ejaculate for over a year.

In females there is delayed puberty*, amenorrhoea* and anovulation*. In young women, low doses of oestradiol* are used to encourage breast development and cyclical oestrogen*/progesterone* preparations are used until fertility treatment is required. HMG* or pulsatile GnRH* therapy will then stimulate ovulation.

Kartagener's syndrome: a structural defect of cilia* throughout the body, resulting in absence or severe impairment of sperm motility, bronchiectasis (chronic lung infection) and chronic sinusitis. There may also be reversal of the internal organs so that the heart is on the right side and the appendix on the left.

karyotype (Fig. 14): a conventional description of the chromosomes* in a cell*, arranged according to their size and centromere* position. A karyotype for a person with Turner's* syndrome, for example, shows only 45 chromosomes, rather than the normal 46.

Klinefelter's syndrome: a congenital disorder occurring in 1 in 1000 males. The men are born with an additional X chromosome* (i.e. XXY). due to abnormal meiosis* during oocyte* development when the two X chromosomes remain in the same oocyte (meiotic non-disjunction*) and do not segregate to two different cells. If the oocyte is fertilized by a Y-bearing chromosome the embryo thus becomes a 47 XXY instead of the normal 46 XY individual.

Affected men are taller than average, thin, with eunuchoid features, female fat distribution, sparse body hair, some breast enlargement and have very small testes*. They are sterile due to azoospermia*, but usually have normal sexual function. There is a deficiency of testosterone* with gross elevation of FSH* and LH* concentrations. In the testes, the seminiferous* tubules are obliterated and men affected by Klinefelter's syndrome are currently incurable and have to consider donor* insemination. Exceptionally (see mosaicism) some areas of spermatogenesis* are seen and pregnancy may then be achieved by TESA* and ICSI*.

Kremer penetration test: a test to study sperm* penetration into cervical* mucus. The mucus is aspirated into a fine capillary tube so that the progress of spermatozoa along the mucus column can be observed microscopically. This is a more sophisticated and accurate type of sperm–cervical mucus contact (SCMC) test, in which the performance of spermatozoa of the male partner can be compared with that of spermatozoa from a fertile donor. Similarly, the ability of the female partner's mid-cycle mucus to permit penetration of her partner's spermatozoa can also be compared with that of mucus obtained from a female of proven fertility. (See sperm–mucus interaction.)

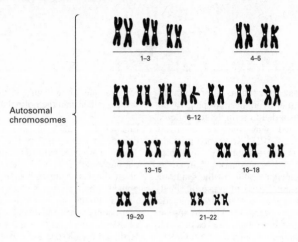

Autosomal chromosomes

1–3   4–5

6–12

13–15   16–18

19–20   21–22

Sex chromosomes

X X   X Y

Fig. **14.** Karotype. A karotype shows the 44 autosomal chromosomes and *either* two X chromosomes (if the person is a female) *or* one X and one Y chromosome (if the person is a male).

L

labia (Fig. 27): the labia majora are two fleshy skin folds which run from the mons pubis (the prominent hair-covered area at the lower end of the abdominal muscles over the junction of the two pubic bones) down to the perineum* (the area between the entrance to the vagina and the anus). They are covered by hair and contain sebaceous and sweat glands. They enclose the labia minora and introitus*.

The labia minora are two delicate thin skin flaps, situated between the labia majora, one on each side of the vaginal opening. They run from the clitoris* above to join in the four-chette* which is continuous with the labia majora and the perineal skin. They are covered by skin on the outer aspect, but by a softer mucous membrane-like epithelium* on the inner aspect. They vary in size, have a rich blood supply and, like the clitoris, are highly sensitive. Between the two labia minora is the introitus* with the vaginal* and urethral* orifices and the opening of the ducts of the Bartholin's* glands.

In the developing male fetus, the labia majora enclose the testes* and fuse to form the scrotum* and the labia minora become fused to form the walls of the penile urethra*.

lactation: term used to refer to both the secretion of milk from the breasts and to breast feeding. The glandular and duct systems of the mammary glands (the breasts) become larger and more active in pregnancy, under the influence of oestrogens* and progesterone*. A yellow, sticky secretion called colostrum* starts appearing in the second half of pregnancy.

The disappearance of oestrogens and progesterone from the maternal blood immediately after delivery allows prolactin* to stimulate the breasts to produce milk. High levels of prolactin (see hyperprolactinaemia) suppress ovarian activity and cause amenorrhoea*. This is the basis for the contraceptive* effect of breast feeding, probably the most widely practised form of female contraception in the world. However, to maintain a high prolactin output, regular stimulation by suckling is necessary and the effectiveness of lactational amenorrhoea* and anovulation*, as a method of birth control, depends not only on the duration of lactation but on the number of feeds given throughout the day and (more important) the night.

laparoscopy (*syn.* coelioscopy or pelviscopy): the technique in which an endoscope* is employed to visualize structures within the peritoneal cavity. The laparoscope consists of a rigid tube with magnifying lenses and uses a cold light source to transmit illumination via bundles of glass fibres. Carbon* dioxide gas is instilled into the abdominal cavity prior to the introduction of the laparoscope.

Originally laparoscopy was used only for diagnostic purposes, for example to establish the patency of the Fallopian* tubes by chromopertubation*, to detect the presence of endometriosis* or to elucidate the cause of pelvic pain. It soon became used for the diagnosis of acute emergencies, for example to differentiate between internal bleeding from a ruptured ovarian cyst* or extra-uterine* pregnancy. Simple laparoscopic operations followed, such as tubal sterilization*, ovarian biopsy* and adhesiolysis*.

Today, the laparoscope is used to perform major operations in both gynaecology and general surgery, a technique known as minimal access, or 'key hole', surgery. In reproductive medicine, the laparoscope is regarded as the 'gold standard' for the diagnosis of pelvic disease. Originally it was used for oocyte* collection in IVF*, but this is now generally performed by the transvaginal route under ultrasound* guidance. It is still used prior to GIFT*. In men, laparoscopic varicocele* ligation can be used as an alternative to open surgery.

Laparoscopy is usually performed under general anaesthesia. Great attention is paid to training in laparoscopy to avoid complications such as perforation of the bowel or internal bleeding.

laparotomy: a surgical incision to gain access to the abdominal cavity in order to inspect the organs within the peritoneal cavity and carry out any necessary operation. General anaesthesia is usually employed.

laser surgery: the term laser is an acronym, derived from the initials of **l**ight **a**mplification by **s**timulated **e**mission of **r**adiation. Lasers produce a highly concentrated beam of light, the energy of which can be used surgically. There are a number of different lasers available for particular surgical procedures such as vaporization (to destroy tissues) and cutting (like a knife through tissues). Laser surgery is relatively bloodless and can be directed towards small lesions without injuring surrounding healthy tissues.

Lasers are used in such widely differing applications as eye surgery and in the treatment of CIN*. In women, laser laparoscopy* can be used in the management of endometriosis*, adhesions*, extra-uterine* pregnancy and distal tubal occlusion (see hydrosalpinx). Laser ablation of the endometrium* can be used in the management of menorrhagia*. In men spot laser welding can be used in microsurgical vasectomy* reversal.

lateral sperm head displacement: a parameter measured in CASA* (computer assisted semen analysis) which is directly related to the fertilizing ability of spermatozoa.

Lesch–Nyhan syndrome: a rare sex-linked*, recessive* congenital abnormality affecting male children; there is an abnormality of purine metabolism which results in mental retardation, cerebral palsy, self-mutilation and early death.

Antenatal diagnosis (chorionic* villus sampling and amniocentesis*) can be used to detect the enzyme* abnormality in families with previously affected offspring. Pre-implantation* diagnostic techniques are being developed.

leiomyoma: see fibroid.

leucorrhoea: *lit.* a white discharge: the term refers to the normal vaginal fluid, comprizing secretions from the cervix and vaginal walls. The discharge is non-irritant and non-offensive, but may vary in amount with different times in the menstrual cycle and is usually heavier in pregnancy.

leukospermia: an increased number of white blood cells in the seminal* fluid, thought to be an indication of infection in the male genital tract.

Leydig cells: the interstitial cells of the testis*, situated between the seminiferous* tubules. They secrete testosterone* in response to pituitary* LH*. Testosterone circulates throughout the body, and high concentrations are maintained within the testis, an essential requirement for spermatogenesis*.

If the seminiferous tubules atrophy* and the testis shrinks, Leydig cells continue to function so that infertile men with azoospermia* or oligozoospermia* due to testicular failure generally do not suffer from testosterone deficiency, and therefore have normal sexual function and secondary sexual* characteristics.

libido: sexual drive or desire. The intensity of libido varies from person to person, and may also vary in women in relation to the menstrual cycle, pregnancy or menopause. Libido generally decreases in both sexes with advancing age. The term must not be confused with orgasm*.

linkage: two or more genes* are said to be linked if they lie on the same chromosome*. The closer together the loci* for the genes are, the tighter they are linked. Closely linked genes tend to be inherited together as the chances of recombination* occurring between them are small. Genes which occur on the X* chromosome are said to be sex-linked*.

liquefaction: immediately after ejaculation*, seminal* fluid coagulates: after this it liquefies (becomes thin) within about 20 minutes. Impaired liquefaction (increased viscosity) may be due to infection in the male accessory* glands, i.e. the seminal* vesicles and prostate* gland.

liquor folliculi: see follicular fluid.

Listeriosis: infection caused by *Listeria monocytogenes*, a Gram negative non-sporing aerobic bacterium* which occurs in many different species, including cattle, pigs, rodents, birds, fish and occasionally humans. The natural habitats of *L. monocytogenes* are soil and decaying vegetable matter, though the organism can be isolated from sewage, water, fresh and frozen poultry, fresh and processed meats, milk and cheese as well as from asymptomatic human and animal carriers.

In non-pregnant adults, *L. monocytogenes* can cause meningitis, encephalitis or septicaemia; these are more common and severe in immuno-compromised patients. In pregnant women, *L. monocytogenes* often causes an influenza-like illness which may infect the fetus, leading to miscarriage*, stillbirth* or premature birth; it is not considered to be a cause of recurrent* miscarriage. Neonates may develop meningo-encephalitis or septicaemia. Listeriosis can occur as sporadic cases or as epidemics; in both, contaminated foods, especially soft cheeses, are usually responsible. Ampicillin is normally an effective treatment.

lithotomy: a term derived from one of the oldest known surgical operations, i.e. cutting for (bladder) stone. It is now used to refer to the position of the patient on the operating table used for many gynaecological procedures such as curettage*, hysteroscopy* and operations on the cervix*. In reproductive medicine the position is used for the transvaginal collection of oocytes and also for embryo* transfer.

In the lithotomy position the patient is placed on the operating table on her back; the hips are flexed with the thighs opened outwards and the legs supported by stirrups attached to poles on the operating table, so that the operator has easy access to the genital tract. The lithotomy position is also used by urologists for endoscopic* procedures on the bladder in both sexes, and by general surgeons or proctologists for operations on the anus and rectum.

live birth rate: the number of infants born alive per 1000 total births. In normal obstetric practice, the live birth rate will be the sum total of babies born per 1000 pregnancies after deducting late miscarriages and stillbirths. In assisted* reproductive technology, the live birth rate is variously calculated per treatment cycle, egg collection, embryo* transfer or pregnancy achieved.

Maternal age*, cause of the infertility and response to treatment protocols will influence the live birth rate, as will the number of abandoned treatment cycles, early LH* surges, failure of fertilization* or cleavage*, failure to implant*, incidence of miscarriage* or extra-uterine* pregnancy. Clinic size and the number of treatment cycles undertaken also influence results.

Variables to be considered in calculating live birth rates include criteria for entry or rejection of patients and criteria for selection of oocytes* and spermatozoa* For these reasons, comparison of results from different clinics is difficult and it is essential to know to which stage in the treatment cycle a reported live birth rate refers.

locus: (*pl.* loci): the place on a chromosome* where a particular gene* is situated.

lupus anticoagulant: this factor is present in the blood of individuals with systemic lupus erythematosus (SLE) and primary anti-phospholipid syndrome. It is responsible for a disorder of blood coagulation and represents an increased risk of both arterial and venous thrombosis*.

Lupus anticoagulant can be an important cause of recurrent* (mainly second trimester*) miscarriages (presumably by compromizing the developing placental* circulation) without the development of SLE itself. Women who suffer from repeated miscarriages and test positive for lupus anticoagulant should be offered low dose aspirin in pregnancy to reduce the likelihood of clot formation. Recent work has shown the additional benefit of heparin in this situation.

Women with a persistently positive lupus test should be advised against using the combined oral contraceptive pills because of the increased risk of thrombosis.

luteal cell: ovarian cell found in the corpus* luteum. The corpus luteum forms from the cells remaining in the follicle* after ovulation*, which become luteinized (*lit.* yellow). These include the granulosa* cells which become granulosa lutein cells, and the theca* cells which become theca lutein cells. The corpus luteum develops a rich blood supply. Both types of luteal cells secrete progesterone* which produces the secretory changes in the endometrium* until the next menstruation or through the first trimester* of pregnancy.

luteal phase (*syn.* secretory phase): the phase in the menstrual cycle from ovulation* to the next menstruation*. During this time, under the influence of progesterone* secreted by the luteal* cells in the corpus* luteum, the endometrium* becomes thicker, more vascular and receptive to a blastocyst* if fertilization* has occurred. The luteal phase usually lasts 14 days and, if it is shorter, this may be a cause of failure of a blastocyst to implant. During the luteal phase, the cervical* mucus becomes thicker and impenetrable to spermatozoa*.

Premenstrual* tension may occur in the late luteal phase, probably caused by increased sensitivity to progesterone secretion.

luteal phase insufficiency: this occurs when ovulation* has taken place, but the corpus* luteum produces insufficient progesterone*: abnormal menstruation may occur, as may failure of implantation* if fertilization* has taken place. Luteal insufficiency is unlikely to be a recurring condition and is no longer considered a cause of recurrent* miscarriage. When it is considered to be associated with infertility, treatment is as for unexplained* infertility.

luteal phase support: this is used in an attempt to improve pregnancy rates in assisted conception cycles where down-regulation has preceded ovarian* stimulation. After embyo transfer*, oral or vaginal progesterone* may be administered daily or low dose hCG* (e.g. 1500 iu) is given every three days for three doses. HCG is not given if there is a significant risk of OHSS*.

There is no clear evidence that giving hCG or progesterone* in the luteal phase improves the outcome in unexplained* infertility or recurrent* miscarriage. (See also ovarian stimulation.)

luteinizing hormone (LH): one of the two gonadotrophins* produced in the anterior lobe of the pituitary* gland under the control of GnRH*. LH is released in a pulsatile manner with the frequency and amplitude varying throughout the menstrual cycle.

A rapid rise (the LH surge) occurs once a threshold concentration of oestradiol* is reached. This is usually on day 12–13 of a 28 day cycle. The LH surge initiates the final stage in the maturation* of the follicle* and oocyte* and leads to ovulation* about 36 to 38 hours after its peak.

LH also has an important role in steroidogenesis*, stimulating androgen* production in the theca* cells during the follicular* phase and progesterone* production in the luteal* phase. Hypersecretion of LH (concentrations greater than 10 iu/L) may occur in women with polycystic* ovarian syndrome and is thought to be associated with infertility* and early pregnancy loss*. Low concentrations of LH (and FSH*) are found in women with amenorrhoea* due to hypothalamic* or pituitary* abnormalities.

In men, pulsatile LH secretion acts on the interstitial (see Leydig*) cells in the testes* and plays a major role in spermatogenesis* and testosterone* production (see gonadotrophins). Low concentrations are found in men with hypogonadotrophic* hypogonadism.

luteinizing hormone releasing hormone (LHRH): see gonadotrophin releasing hormone (GnRH).

luteinized unruptured follicle (LUF): a condition where the follicle* matures but does not rupture. Despite this failure of ovulation, the theca* and granulosa* cells are luteinized and serum progesterone* concentrations rise in the luteal* phase. Hormonal changes are therefore of little help in establishing the diagnosis which is made by serial ultrasound* scanning of the ovaries or by observing their condition at laparoscopy*.

The clinical significance of the LUF syndrome is doubtful as the condition is probably an occasional event and does not recur in subsequent menstrual cycles.

M

Makler chamber: a laboratory device to facilitate microscopic semen* analysis. It consists of a thin flat chamber, 10 microns deep with a visible lattice dividing the surface into squares. Sperm concentration and motility can be assessed rapidly. The motility characteristics can be analysed by time-lapse photography or a computerized technique.

male accessory glands: see accessory glands.

male genital tract (Fig. 15): this comprises the testis*, epididymis*, vas deferens*, ejaculatory* ducts, accessory* glands and urethra*.

male subfertility: failure of a couple to conceive due to impaired fertility of the male partner. This may be due to abnormalities of the semen* or spermatozoa*, or mechanical factors that interfere with sperm deposition at the female's external cervical* os, for example: low semen volume, hypospadias*, impotence*, retrograde* ejaculation or ejaculation* failure due to spinal* cord injury.

Semen abnormalities include azoospermia*, sperm coating due to anti-sperm* antibodies and subnormal semen quality (see oligospermia, oligozoospermia, asthenozoospermia and oligoasthenoteratozoospermia).

The majority of subfertile men have subnormal semen quality of unknown origin. Many men with apparently normal semen have unexplained infertility because their spermatozoa cannot fertilize (see sperm* dysfunction).

MAR test: mixed antiglobulin reaction test. A routine screening* test for antisperm* antibodies, similar to the immunobead test. (See immunobead test.)

marsupialisation: a surgical technique in which a cyst is everted rather than excised. This is particularly used in the management of Bartholin's* cysts and makes the operation quicker and more bloodless than excision of the gland; it also reduces the incidence of recurrence.

mastalgia: pain in the breasts. This is common at puberty* in boys as well as girls. In women it mainly occurs premenstrually, in early pregnancy and in the fourth and fifth decades when the condition is often referred to as

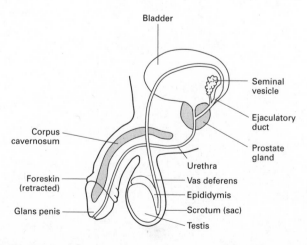

Fig. **15**. The Male Genital Tract.

chronic mastitis and is associated with nodularity and cystic dilatation of ducts and gland tissue. It is thought that premenstrual mastalgia only occurs in cycles in which ovulation* has occurred and that it is associated with changing progesterone* concentrations. Mastalgia may also occur, particularly initially, with the use of combined oral contraceptive* pills and hormone* replacement therapy.

maternal age: see age.

maternal mortality: see mortality rates.

maturation: in oocytes* this is the progression through meiosis* from prophase I (the germinal* vesicle stage, immature) to metaphase II (mature). Mature oocytes at metaphase II are ready for ovulation* and fertilization*. Maturation is stimulated *in vivo* by the midcycle luteinizing* hormone surge (LH surge), or by an injection of human* chorionic gonadotrophin (hCG). Maturation of human oocytes may occur *in vitro*, but, with present techniques, such oocytes are usually less fertile than those matured *in vivo*.

In spermatogenesis*, spermatogonia* undergo meiosis* and mature through primary and secondary spermatocyte* stages into spermatids* which elongate and develop tails to become spermatozoa*. Maturation arrest can occur at any of these stages; its aetiology is generally uncertain, although some cases are due to genetic* disorders.

The term sperm maturation also refers to the process whereby the spermatozoa, passing through the epididymis*, develop their motility and fertilizing ability.

The term maturation also applies to the stage in adolescence* in both sexes when the changes of puberty* are completed and procreation is possible. Emotional and intellectual changes accompany the physical changes, but take longer to complete.

mean value: a phrase generally used to denote the arithmetic mean value or average*, which in a sample of observations is simply the sum of the observations divided by the number in the sample. Mean value coincides with the median* and the mode for symmetrical distributions.

meconium: the content of the fetal bowel. It is greenish in colour, sterile and highly viscous and consists of bile salts, cellular debris, vernix (the sebaceous covering of the fetal skin *in utero*) and other substances present in the amniotic* fluid and swallowed by

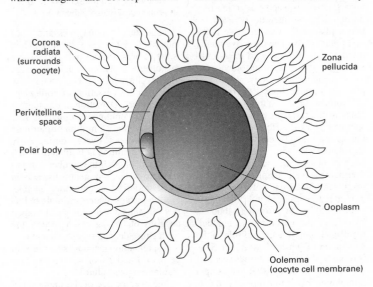

Corona radiata (surrounds oocyte)

Zona pellucida

Perivitelline space

Polar body

Ooplasm

Oolemma (oocyte cell membrane)

Fig. **17**. Mature Human Oocyte.

the fetus. Passage of meconium into the amniotic* fluid in pregnancy or labour may be a sign of fetal distress occasioned by lack of oxygen.

median: the central value of a sample, or of a distribution, so that 50% of the sample/distribution lies below the median value and 50% above the median value. The median is a useful statistic for asymmetric distributions. It coincides with the mean* for symmetric distributions.

medium: see culture medium.

medroxyprogesterone: an injectable, long-acting progestogen* which suppresses ovulation* and is used for contraception* and occasionally in the treatment of endometriosis*. It is given at three monthly intervals. Menstrual irregularity may be associated with its use.

meiosis: cell division in which a diploid* cell with 46 chromosomes* divides twic , to give rise to four 'daughter' cells each with the haploid* number of 23 chromosomes.

Meiosis takes place only in the formation of the gametes, i.e. oocytes* and spermatozoa*. Oocytes are formed in the ovaries* by the process of oogenesis*. Here diploid precursor cells undergo meiosis, each one giving rise, during the first meiotic division, to two haploid cells. One of these is the first polar* body. The other eventually divides, during the second meiotic division, to give rise to an oocyte and to a second polar body. (See also maturation, polar body.) Spermatozoa are formed in the seminiferous* tubules of the testes* by the process of spermatogenesis*. Here diploid spermatogonial* stem* cells give rise to spermatocytes* which undergo meiosis, each one giving rise to four haploid spermatozoa. The haploid cells that result from meiosis, only have their diploid nature restored at fertilization*.

In addition to bringing about a halving of the chromosome number, meiosis also plays a central role in the generation of genetic* variation. This is brought about partly because each of the two chromosomes that makes up a homologous* pair in a diploid cell carries different alleles*. As a result, the haploid cells that result from meiosis are bound to be different from one another. Furthermore, the different pairs of homologous chromosomes separate entirely independently of each other, so that the daughter cells end up containing different combinations of chromosomes. A further reason why meiosis promotes genetic variation is that it involves the formation of chiasmata*— sites at which genetic material is exchanged between chromatids*. (See also mitosis.)

membrana granulosa: see granulosa cell.

menarche: the age at which menstruation* first occurs. This is the most definite sign (though not necessarily the first) that puberty* has commenced. Over the last 100 years, the average age of the menarche has steadily declined in the Western world from the age of 14 to 16 years to between 12 and 13 years. This change is probably related to better nutrition and increased body weight in adolescents. Conversely the menarche is delayed in girls suffering from malnutrition Contrary to common belief, the age of the menarche is not related to climate. The onset of menstruation does not directly equate with the onset of fertility as the early menstrual cycles in adolescents are often anovular*. (See also puberty.)

menopause: *lit.* the cessation of monthly periods. Just as the menarche* is the clearest sign of puberty*, so the menopause is the most definitive sign of the climacteric*. The menopause is caused by cessation of follicular* development. Depletion in the number of oocytes* continues throughout life: there are about 3.5 million primordial* follicles in each ovary* during early fetal life, 1 million at birth and 10 000 by the age of 40. If the number drops to 1000 or below, the menopause sets in as oestradiol* concentrations decline. Fertility drugs cannot stimulate further follicular development and women desirous of having children after the menopause depend on egg* donation.

A premature menopause occurs in between 1 and 2% of women (see premature ovarian failure).

The average age of the menopause, within a given population, is more variable than that of the menarche*, normally between 45 and 54 years (averaging 51.8 years in the UK). It varies with familial, racial and nutritional factors.

At the climacteric, different changes of menstrual patterns are experienced by different women, such as abrupt cessation of the menses, regular but scantier menstruation, heavier menstrual losses or prolonged intervals between menstrual periods.

Significant physical and emotional changes may precede, accompany or follow the menopause. Hormone* replacement therapy (HRT) can correct many of these changes, which include hot flushes, night sweats, mood swings, depression, irritability, bladder problems, vaginal dryness during intercourse, and, in the long run, osteoporosis* and heart disease. Oestrogen* therapy is the mainstay of treatment, but, to protect the endometrium* from the development of cancer, the addition of progestogens* is required in women who have not had a hysterectomy*.

menorrhagia: unduly heavy or prolonged menstrual losses at normal intervals. This may be associated with uterine abnormalities such as submucous fibroids*, endometrial polyps* or adenomyosis*, endocrine* disorders such as hypothyroidism* or there may be no detectable cause in which case the condition is labelled 'dysfunctional uterine bleeding'. Social, psychosexual and emotional factors may play a role. For research purposes, menorrhagia is defined as a blood loss of more than 80 ml in the course of one menstruation.

menstruation: the shedding of the endometrium* consequent on the falling oestrogen* and progesterone* concentrations at the end of the luteal* phase of the menstrual* cycle. The endometrium regenerates and thickens in the proliferative* phase of the cycle, becomes more active and vascular in the secretory (luteal) phase and is discarded as the menstrual loss if implantation* has not occurred. If implantation has occurred, the corpus* luteum continues to produce oestradiol* and progesterone*, menstruation is suppressed and the endometrium becomes decidualized*. (See menstrual cycle.)

menstrual cycle: the rhythmicity of menstruation* which is controlled by the secretion of the pituitary gonadotrophins* which in turn stimulate the ovaries* to produce oestrogens* and progesterone* and control the phases of the cycle. When serum concentrations of these hormones decline, endometrial* shedding is initiated and the menstrual loss consists of endometrial glands and secretions as well as blood.

The length of a menstrual cycle is counted in days from the first day of one period to the first day of the next. The average duration is 28 days, but variations of 24 to 35 days are accepted as within normal limits. Cycles shorter or longer than this are more likely to be anovulatory*. The duration of the menstrual flow is very variable and whilst the average is 3 to 5 days, durations of 1 to 8 days can be normal. Equally variable is the amount of the menstrual loss, but more than 80 ml is considered excesssive (see menorrhagia).

The phases of the menstrual cycle may be monitored by basal* body temperature recordings, ultrasound* scans or serum hormone* concentrations. This is of particular importance for the correct timing of oocyte collection in IVF* and of artificial* insemination. In ART* the natural menstrual cycle may be replaced by stimulated cycles (see ovarian stimulation) to produce more oocytes*, or may be manipulated to induce ovulation* on a fixed day, for example in relation to egg* donation. (See also endometrium, gonadotrophins.)

menstrual disorders: these include menorrhagia*, hypomenorrhoea*, polymenorrhoea*, oligomenorrhoea* and amenorrhoea*. Dysmenorrhoea* and premenstrual* tension are common and indicate that ovulation* has occurred and progesterone* concentrations are raised.

MESA (microsurgical epididymal sperm aspiration, Fig. 24): a method of surgical collection of spermatozoa* carried out in cases of irreversible obstructive* azoospermia. Usually performed under general anaesthesia, sperm-containing fluid is aspirated from a microscopically incised tubule on the surface of the epididymis*. The epididymal tubules are then repaired microsurgically*. Aspirated spermatozoa are used for ICSI* and any surplus is cryopreserved*.

MESA is mainly indicated when sperm collection for ICSI is combined with microsurgical reconstructive procedures. Otherwise, spermatozoa adequate for ICSI can be collected more rapidly and economically by needle aspiration of the epididymis (PESA) under local anaesthesia.

mesosalpinx (Fig. 8): the flimsy peritoneal fold which is attached to the lower border of the Fallopian* tube and runs to the ovary*. This is a highly vascular and pliable structure. In pelvic* inflammatory disease it is particularly likely to be involved, leading to its occlusion with resultant adhesions* between tube and ovary and interference with tubal motility. Re-opening of the mesosalpinx is performed in microsurgery* in order to restore normal anatomy and tubal mobility.

mesterolone (Proviron): a synthesized compound with androgenic* activity used in the treatment of male subfertility, but with no proven beneficial effect.

meta-analysis: a relatively new statistical term used to describe an investigation where the results of several independent studies are combined to provide a single composite finding. Although the method is appealing when applied to all the studies carried out by one researcher or laboratory, its application to a batch of results obtained from published papers is more problematical and controversial. Publication bias, a well documented phenomenon whereby papers reporting positive findings are more likely to be published than those with inconclusive findings, would tend to distort the composite finding.

metaphase: the stage in both meiosis* and mitosis* when the chromosomes* arrange themselves on a spindle, preparatory to anaphase*.

methotrexate: a synthetic drug which is a folic* acid antagonist. Large amounts of folic acid are required for normal placental* development and the administration of methotrexate in early pregnancy interferes with this. It is used by local injection for the treatment of unruptured tubal pregnancy (see extra-uterine pregnancy) and by the oral route for the treatment of choriocarcinoma*. This is a cytotoxic drug with potential hazards and it should only be used by doctors with special experience.

Methotrexate is occasionally used in the treatment of psoriasis and can impair spermatogenesis*.

microsurgical epididymal sperm aspiration: see MESA.

micro-injection (Fig. 1): a technique to insert spermatozoa* into oocytes* by micromanipulation* in vitro. This is used in couples with poor quality semen* or previous fertilization failure. In subzonal* insemination (SUZI), several spermatozoa are injected under the zona* pellucida, whereas in intracytoplasmic* sperm injection (ICSI), a single spermatozoon is injected directly into the cytoplasm* of the oocyte. The superior fertilization and pregnancy rates following ICSI have reduced the usefulness of SUZI.

micromanipulation: use of apparatus which scales down the movements of the operator's hands. The apparatus facilitates very delicate procedures, such as injection of individual spermatozoa* into oocytes*, or removal of single cells from embryos, using pipettes only a few thousandths of a millimetre thick. The techniques are also used in microsurgical procedures in the male reproductive tract, for example spot laser welding and MESA*.

microsurgery: the surgical technique used in the management of delicate structures where precision and attention to minutiae are of paramount importance. Respect for the tissues and their gentle handling is the over-riding principle. This is achieved by the use of special fine instruments, atraumatic teflon retracting rods, ultra-fine non-reactive suture materials and scrupulous arrest of any bleeding points. Special magnifying glasses (operating loupes) or an operating microscope may be employed. All tissue trauma is avoided as far as possible by gentle handling, keeping the operative field moist and refraining from the use of rough swabs or hot packs.

In tubal surgery the aim of the operator is to restore normal anatomy, perform adhesiolysis* and carry out any necessary procedure such as dealing with a tubal occlusion. Success in restoring fertility depends on the severity of tubal damage, the extent of any adhesions present, the techniques employed and the expertise of the operator.

In the management of male infertility, microsurgical techniques are used in obstructive* azoospermia to by-pass epididymal* obstruction by epididymo-vasotomy*, in reversal of vasectomy* and for MESA*.

Similar surgical techniques are employed in other branches of surgery, such as vascular, plastic and neuro-surgery.

midcycle: the time in the menstrual* cycle when ovulation* is expected to occur. In a 28 day cycle this is usually around day 13 or 14.

midcycle mucus: see cervical mucus. Awareness of the increase in the quantity and fluidity of the cervical mucus at midcycle* is used by some women as an aid to enhancing the prospects of conception* (the fertile period) or for contraception* by avoiding intercourse at this time (the safe period).

mid-luteal progesterone measurement: the serum progesterone* concentration is raised in the secretory phase of the menstrual* cycle after ovulation* has occurred. In the average 28 day cycle, the serum progesterone concentration is measured on day 21. If a patient has regular longer cycles, the test is performed 7 days before the next expected menstruation, for example on day 26 if a patient has 33 day cycles. If cycles are irregular, serial measurements can be done. If a cycle has been monitored by ultrasound, the date of ovulation should be known and the test is performed 7 days after ovulation.

Serum progesterone concentrations greater than 30 nmol/l are taken as evidence of ovulation. If the next expected period is delayed and the progesterone concentration remains high, an early pregnancy is virtually certain.

mifepristone (RU 486): a synthetic progesterone* antagonist, used in the medical termination of pregnancy. In the UK, mifepristone can only be prescribed in a licensed hospital and by a 'recognized' doctor. Women return to hospital 36 to 48 hours after taking the tablets for the administration of intra-vaginal prostaglandins* and miscarriage usually occurs within eight hours.

miscarriage (*syn*. abortion): the spontaneous loss of a pregnancy before the 24th week of pregnancy. Spontaneous miscarriage is very common: at least 15 to 20% of all conceptions miscarry and 95% of these do so in the first trimester. The above figures refer to clinically diagnosed pregnancies: the actual number of conceptions (as demonstrated by an early rise in β hCG pregnancy* tests) that miscarry is much higher.

Clinical types: a miscarriage is 'threatened' when bleeding has occurred but there are no uterine contractions and the cervical* os remains closed; it is 'inevitable' when the bleeding is accompanied by painful contractions and cervical dilatation*; 'complete' when the product of conception have all been expelled; 'incomplete' when the fetus has been expelled and placental tissue remains in the uterus; 'septic' when associated with uterine infection; 'missed' when the fetal sac is intact with or without a non-viable fetus, but is not expelled.

Spontaneous miscarriages, if sporadic, are commonly associated with genetic abnormalities, infections or hormonal factors; if recurrent, causes include abnormalities of the uterus (malformations), cervical* incompetence, immunological and hormonal factors. (See recurrent miscarriage.)

mitochondria: microscopic structures (organelles) that are present in the cytoplasm* of every cell* and which control energy generation by respiration. Large numbers of mitochondria are present in the cytoplasm* of oocytes* and also in the midpiece of spermatozoa* where they are essential for sperm motility.

mitosis: cell division in which a cell*

retains, rather than halves, its chromosome* complement. In humans, mitosis occurs in diploid* cells. Indeed, all the diploid cells an adult human has are the result of successive mitotic cell divisions from the original single zygote* formed at fertilization*.

Mitosis also plays an important role in the repair of the body. For example, new surface skin cells are continually made as a result of mitosis occurring in the underlying cells. Most human cells divide by mitosis. Exceptions include cells which lack a nucleus* (e.g. red blood cells), mature nerve cells and the germ* cells which give rise to oocytes* and spermatozoa* as a result of meiosis*. As cells divide by mitosis, various changes in their genetic make-up gradually accumulate and it is these which can eventually lead to a person's old age and death.

mittelschmerz: *lit.* pain in the middle: lower abdominal pain in women which occurs at mid-cycle* and is generally assumed to be associated with ovulation*. It is suggested that the pain is due to peritoneal irritation by follicular fluid and blood following rupture of the follicle*. However, the relation of the pain to the exact time of ovulation and to the side on which ovulation has occurred is variable.

mole: see hydatidiform mole.

mongolism: see Down's syndrome.

moniliasis: see *Candida albicans*.

monosomy: abnormal genetic make-up in which one of the chromosomes* is missing so that a cell has only 45 instead of 46 chromosomes. With the exception of Turner's* syndrome, in which the woman concerned has just a single X chromosome, monosomy is fatal and almost always results in miscarriage* early in pregnancy.

monozygotic twins (uniovular twins): identical twins* resulting from the splitting of an early embryo* created by the fertilization of a single oocyte* by a single spermatozoon*. Monozygotic twins are of the same sex, are genetically identical and usually share a common placenta*. It is not known what causes splitting of the embryo, but physical constriction of the embryo during hatching* might be a causative factor. In animals, deliberate splitting of the pre-implantation embryo by micromanipulation* procedures can result in identical twins.

In humans, splitting can occur up to day 14 of embryonic development. Incomplete splitting will result in the formation of conjoined twins. (See multiple pregnancy.)

morphology: the science and study of form and shape in living organisms. For example, in women, the morphology of the uterus is of significance for reproduction. Abnormal uterine morphology is usually the result of fusion failures of the Müllerian* ducts and can lead to problems with conception*, or cause miscarriage* or labour complications.

In men, the morphology of spermatozoa* is a useful indicator of their fertilizing ability, and may therefore serve as a test of sperm function. If less than 30% of spermatozoa are normal, there is a high chance of fertilization failure in routine IVF* practice and thus a strong indication for ICSI*.

mortality rates:

Maternal: the number of women dying in pregnancy, at delivery or in the 6 weeks after delivery, per 100 000 deliveries. 'Direct' deaths are those resulting from obstetric complications: the principal of these are thrombosis* and embolism*, hypertensive* disorders, haemorrhage, extra-uterine* pregnancy and sepsis. 'Indirect' deaths are those resulting from pre-existing disease or disease developed during pregnancy and not due to direct obstetric causes, but aggravated by the physiological effects of pregnancy, such as heart disease.

In the UK the number of obstetric deaths has decreased dramatically from 70/100 000 in the early 1950s to about 5.5 /100 000 in the late 1990s. The maternal mortality rate is very much higher in many developing countries and is a sensitive index of not only the quality of maternity care, but also of general living standards and the place of women in society. In the UK, *Reports on Confidential Enquiries into Maternal Deaths* are published every 3 years. They analyse the causes of maternal deaths, determine cases of substandard care and make recommendations for management.

Stillbirth: the stillbirth rate is the number of babies born dead after the 24th week of pregnancy per 1000 deliveries. Causes of stillbirth include fetal abnormalities, pre-eclampsia* and eclampsia, diabetes*, ante-partum haemorrhage, umbilical* cord complications, ante-partum anoxia and birth trauma.

Neonatal: the number of children born alive and dying within 28 days per 1000 live births. This is subdivided into perinatal deaths—the number of stillbirths and first week neonatal deaths—and those dying in the rest of the neonatal period. The reason for this distinction is that the main causes for stillbirth and death in the first week of life are related to obstetric factors. Deaths in the rest of the neonatal period are related to more general factors such as infections, accidents and (in some parts of the world) malnutrition. In the UK, the perinatal mortality rate (PNMR) in the 1990s is approximately 8/1000.

The infant mortality rate is the number of infants per 1000 live births who die between the second and twelfth month of life.

All these mortality rates reflect environmental factors, such as social and economic trends, as much as the quality of medical care.

morula: compacted pre-implantation embryo* usually containing approximately 16 cells in humans, evident on days 3–4 after insemination. The morula appears as a solid cluster, in which individual cells cannot be distinguished. Formation of the blastocele* cavity has not yet begun.

mosaicism: the coexistence of genetically different cell populations within a single individual. Mosaicism differs from chimaerism* in that the individual arises from a single zygote*. Mosaicism may occur naturally, e.g. random X-inactivation in females causes two cell populations depending on which X chromosome is inactivated. Similarly, mutation* of a gene* during development may give rise to daughter cells which are different from unmutated neighbouring cells. Such mutations may also be induced experimentally in animals as a research procedure, or new genes can be injected (see transgenics). These techniques can provide important information on the fate of individual cells whose progeny can be mapped through later stages of development.

Mosaicism occurs occasionally in men with Klinefelter's* syndrome (XXY) who may then have spermatozooa* in the semen* or, if azoospermic*, foci of normal functioning XY seminiferous* tubules in the testes* from which spermatozoa can be retrieved for ICSI*.

Müllerian duct: the embryonic (paramesonephric) ducts which first appear in the 10 mm embryo and, in the female, form the Fallopian* tubes, uterus* and upper vagina*. The upper ends of the ducts remain open as the trumpet-shaped abominal openings (infundibulum*) of the tubes. The lower ends fuse with each other to form (in humans) the single cavity uterus, cervix and upper vagina.

Failure of fusion (Fig. 16), if complete, can produce duplication of the uterus and vagina (see didelphys uterus), whilst lesser degrees of fusion failure, which are relatively common, produce anomalies such as a bicornuate* uterus or vaginal septum.

multiple pregnancy: a pregnancy in which two or more fetuses co-exist in the uterus. The majority of multiple pregnancies are twin pregnancies: higher order pregnancies are progressively rarer. The majority of twin pregnancies (about 75%) are dizygotic* (binovular) and result in the birth of non-identical twins who have separate placentas, can be of different sex and resemble each other no more than other siblings. Both genetic and environmental factors operate in the causation of dizygotic twins. About 25% of twins are monozygotic* (uniovular): they are of the same sex, genetically identical and usually share a common placenta. It is not known what causes monozygotic twinning (see monozygotic twins).

The incidence of multiple pregnancy is much higher during early embryonic development than at delivery. Ultrasound* scanning has shown that there

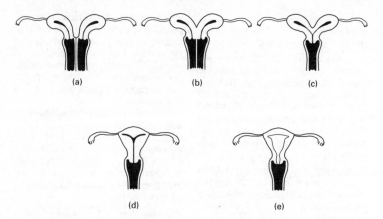

Fig. 16. Müllerian Duct Fusion Abnnormalities. Illustration showing some of the commoner fusion defects:

(a) Uterus didelphys with double vagina   (b) Bicornuate uterus with septate vagina
(c) Bicornate uterus with normal vagina   (d) Subseptate uterus.
(e) Normal uterus with normal vagina.

are frequently two embryonic sacs, but only one may contain a fetus. Loss of the second sac may be associated with a small vaginal bleed and diagnosed as a threatened* miscarriage. Absorption of the second sac without any bleeding is known as the 'vanishing fetus' syndrome. Overall, the incidence of twinning at delivery after spontaneous conception* is about 1:80, of triplets about 1:8000, of quadruplets about 1:400 000 and of quintuplets about 1:40 million births. There are wide regional variations and, for example, in some African countries the incidence of twinning is as high as 1 in 22. The chance of having twins also increases with advancing maternal age.

Multiple pregnancy is associated with many minor and major complications in pregnancy and at delivery. By far the most serious of these are miscarriage*, prematurity* and the delivery of very low birth-weight infants. This hazard increases in direct relation to the degree of multiple pregnancy.

The incidence of multiple pregnancy is greatly increased after ovarian* stimulation. Very high order multiple pregnancies (up to eight fetuses) have occurred following ovulation induction in women with infertility, particularly in the management of amenorrhoea*. In IVF*, transfer of more than one embryo* increases the pregnancy rate and

in the early days of IVF treatment, large numbers of embryos were sometimes transferred in order to achieve a pregnancy. This resulted in a high incidence of multiple pregnancies. Most multiple pregnancies following ovarian stimulation and IVF and ET* are of non-identical embryos as expected following the maturation of several follicles* and the transfer of several embryos into one patient. For reasons not known there is, however, also an increased incidence of identical twinning after IVF.

Realisation of the physical and emotional risks of a high order multiple pregnancy, including a high risk of miscarriage or extreme prematurity, has led to the use of fetal* reduction. The Code of Practice of the HFEA* now limits the number of embryos that may be transferred after IVF to 2 or, at the most, 3. Even such limitation still produces a multiple pregnancy rate of about 25%. Ovulation induction, including superovulation and intra-uterine* insemination (IUI), without IVF is not controlled by the HFEA*. Careful monitoring of follicular development is required in these cases. Cycles should be abandoned if more than three follicles have been stimulated.

mumps: a common childhood infection, presenting with swelling and tenderness of one or both parotid glands. When this infection occurs in post-pubertal men, 20 to 30% suffer epididymo-orchitis* at the time of, or soon after, the parotid swelling. This complication affects both testicles* in only one in six cases. Significant swelling and inflammation* of the testicle occur and normally resolve spontaneously within a week or so. Some atrophy* can occur in the affected testis. Inevitably this condition causes considerable anxiety, though few patients develop secondary infertility, even if both testes were affected.

Oophoritis* and first trimester* miscarriage* are rare complications of mumps infection in women.

mutation: the inherited change to genetic material. Gene* mutations involve a change within just a single gene. Chromosome* mutations involve greater structural changes including the gain or loss of entire chromosomes.

mycoplasma: tiny free-living organisms commonly found in the female genital tract. Some investigators have suggested an association between the presence of mycoplasma and various reproductive problems including miscarriage*, premature delivery and growth retardation in babies. However, the weight of scientific evidence is against any major effect.

myoma: see fibroid.

myomectomy: the surgical operation at which one or more fibroids* are removed, without removing the uterus*. Such a procedure can be more difficult technically and involve greater blood loss than a hysterectomy*. Pre-operatively, GnRH* analogues can be used to reduce the size of the fibroids and their blood supply and thus make the operation easier.

The removal of subserous and intramural fibroids (see Fig. 10) usually requires a laparotomy*. Good haemostasis and meticulous surgical technique are required to prevent post-operative adhesion* formation. Laparoscopic* myomectomy is sometimes performed in preference to an open operation, but haemostasis can be difficult. Hysteroscopic* myomectomy can be used for the removal of submucous fibroids.

Myomectomy is only performed in women who wish to retain their reproductive capacity. Growth of further fibroids may occur after myomectomy and this has to be clearly explained to patients. In women complaining of infertility, in whom asymptomatic intramural fibroids are found, and where there are no other infertility factors, myomectomy is sometimes followed by conception*.

myometrium: the bundles of non-striated (smooth) muscle fibres which constitute the substance of the uterus*. These muscle fibres are capable of enormous increase in size and number during pregnancy to contain the growing fetus. In labour, the muscle fibres not only contract but also retract, i.e. remain permanently shortened. This leads to the taking up and dilatation of the cervix* and eventually the delivery of the fetus.

myxoedema: the clinical syndrome associated with deficiency of thyroid* hormone (hypothyroidism*) in the adult. Typical features include a pale, dry and coarse skin, weight gain, mental slowness and cold intolerance. In women there may be irregular and heavy menstruation, amenorrhoea* or ovulation* failure. Men may become impotent*. Treatment with thyroxine needs to be life long and reverses all the symptoms.

N

Nabothian follicle: small retention cyst*, visible and palpable on the external* cervical os . These cysts result from obstruction of the ducts of cervical glands and may be one of the features of chronic cervicitis*. They do not require treatment.

natural killer cells: cells which are a subset of lymphocytes (one type of the white blood corpuscles) and play a role in the early, non-specific phases of the immune* response. The cells do not recognize foreign antigens* as such but, once activated by cytokines*, may kill cells with abnormal signals present on their surface. Natural killer cells are present in the endometrium* of the uterus and it has been suggested that they may play a role in recurrent* miscarriages, though the evidence for this is far from conclusive.

necrozoospermia: spermatozoa* in which no motility is observed. This may be due to structural defects of the sperm tail, detectable by electron microscopy. (See also immotile cilia syndrome.)

Neisseria: a genus of bacteria* which includes the organism that causes gonorrhoea*. The term is sometimes used loosely, and incorrectly, to mean gonorrhoea.

neonate: the baby in the first month of life.

neonatal mortality rate: the number of babies born alive and dying in the first month of life per 1000 total live births. (See mortality rates.)

neosalpingostomy: see salpingostomy.

Neubauer chamber: a microscope slide designed for counting red blood cells. It has been adapted for use in the measurement of sperm* numbers (density) and is a device similar to, but less informative than, the Makler* chamber. In assisted conception and andrology* clinics, the Makler chamber has gained wider acceptance, whilst in general hospitals and pathology departments the improved Neubauer haematocytometer is used more frequently for semen* analysis.

neural tube defect: congenital abnormalities affecting the bones of the skull and spine. The term includes anencephaly* (which is incompatible with life) and spina* bifida where there is a closure defect of the spine, so that parts of the spinal cord, brain tissue or their covering membranes protrude. Degrees of spina bifida vary from the minor, asymptomatic to major which may cause death or severe disability. There are marked regional and seasonal variations in the incidence of neural tube defects. Together they constitute one of the commonest forms of fetal malformation and an important factor in perinatal mortality*.

Antenatal screening with alphafeto* protein (AFP) estimations and ultrasound* can detect most neural tube defects in pregnancy and, in some cases, may provide an indication to terminate pregnancy. The incidence of neural tube defects is reduced by the administration of folic* acid prior to conception* and in early pregnancy. This should be prescribed for all women, but particularly those with a previous affected baby. (See also anencephaly, spina bifida, folic acid.)

non-disjunction: a mistake during meiosis* which causes some resulting haploid* cells to have only 22 chromosomes* and others 24 chromosomes, instead of the normal 23. If a gamete* with 22 chromosomes fuses with one with the normal 23, a zygote* with 45 chromosomes results (monosomy*). If a gamete with 24 chromosomes fuses with one with 23, a zygote with 47 results (trisomy*).

non-specific urethritis (NSU): a sexually* transmitted disease, caused by *Chlamydia* trachomatis*. Infected men have a burning pain when passing urine and usually a scanty green penile discharge. There is a very high risk of transmission to the female partner in whom symptoms vary from minimal to severe. Treatment with antibiotics should be prescribed for both partners. In men, NSU can lead to prostatitis* and/or epididymitis* which may be followed by obstructive* azoospermia. (See also *Chlamydia trachomatis*, pelvic inflammatory disease, salpingitis, sexually transmitted diseases.)

norethisterone: a synthetic progestogen* widely used in gynaecology, for oral contraception*, hormone* replacement therapy and the management of dysfunctional uterine bleeding (see menorrhagia). In ovarian* stimulation, it can be used to programme treatment cycles. In many oral contraceptive pills, norethisterone has been replaced by newer progestogens*.

nucleic acid: a class of biochemical compounds made up of chains of nucleotides, each nucleotide containing a characteristic five-carbon sugar, a phosphate group and one of a number of possible nitrogenous bases. There are two classes of nucleic acids: deoxyribonucleic acid (DNA*), the genetic material of almost all organisms, and ribonucleic acid (RNA*) which, in most cells, serves to make proteins* from the instructions coded in DNA.

nucleolus (Fig. 3): the region of the cell nucleus* where ribosomal RNA* is synthesized. Nucleoli have a characteristic appearance, usually darker than the rest of the nucleus. There can be up to about 5 nucleoli in each cell nucleus.

nucleus (Fig. 3): the membrane-bound, spherical part of the cell* which contains the chromosomes* and which controls virtually all the activities of the cell. Almost all cells have a nucleus: exceptions include red blood cells and viruses.

O

obesity: weight more than 20% above average in an individual relating to his/her height, due to excessive fat deposition. In obese women amenorrhoea* and other menstrual disturbances are common and obesity is particularly (though not invariably) associated with polycystic* ovarian syndrome. FSH* concentrations may be low and an inadequate luteal* phase is common. Obesity may seriously affect reproductive performance and increase the risk of miscarriage*, but many obese women remain fertile.

In most overweight men, fertility is normal, but in the grossly obese, the number and motility of spermatozoa* may be impaired. This is probably due to excessive fat deposition in the pubic area leading to increased testicular* temperature.

obstructive azoospermia: infertility due to bilateral obstructions in the male* genital tract (Fig. 15), preventing the passage of spermatozoa* into the semen*, seen in about 1% of infertile men. Testicular* size, sperm production, serum FSH* and testosterone* concentrations are all normal.

The obstruction may occur at any site in the male reproductive system. Common causes are bilateral congenital absence of the vas* deferens (BCAV), post-inflammatory epididymal* obstruction and previous vasectomy*. Surgical* sperm retrieval (see epididymal sperm aspiration) for ICSI* is required for treatment of BCVA. Reconstructive surgery is performed in other cases with a good chance of success, but if this fails, surgical sperm retrieval for ICSI* can still be undertaken.

oestradiol (E₂): a sex steroid* hormone*, 90% of which is produced by the developing follicles* in ovulatory women under the influence of FSH*.

Androgens* are converted to oestradiol by the enzyme* aromatase in the granulosa* cells of the dominant follicle and, after ovulation*, in the corpus* luteum.

Increasing amounts of oestradiol are produced at puberty*, leading to the development of the secondary sexual* characteristics which include breast development, growth of pubic hair, maturation of the genital tract and female fat distribution. Oestradiol promotes proliferation of the endometrium* and together with progesterone* produces secretory endometrium. Decreases in oestradiol and progesterone induce menstruation*. Lack of oestradiol from the dominant follicle causes amenorrhoea* and failure of endometrial development.

Oestradiol also has other widespread functions in women's metabolism, including bone deposition and relaxation of smooth muscle of the coronary arteries. After the menopause*, there may be an increased incidence of osteoporosis* and coronary heart disease.

In assisted conception techniques, gonadotrophin* therapy leads to the growth of multiple ovarian follicles; this is reflected in a rise of oestradiol concentrations and is used to monitor treatment. Approximately 500 pmol/l oestradiol are produced per developing follicle. The endometrial thickness reflects the concentrations of oestradiol and can be used for ultrasound* monitoring of stimulated cycles.

oestriol (E₃): an oestrogen* produced by the placenta*, the precursor for which comes from the fetal adrenal* glands and liver. Concentrations of oestriol can thus be used to monitor the well-being of a pregnancy.

oestrogens: a group of C18 sex steroid* hormones* including oestrone (E₁)*, oestradiol* (E₂) and oestriol* (E₃). Oestrogens are produced in various tissues in both men and women from conversion of androgens*. Women produce large quantities of oestradiol from the ovaries, and this is the main feminizing hormone.

Natural and synthetic oestrogens are used in the treatment of amenorrhoea* and other menstrual* disorders. They form part of the combined oral contraceptive* pill, are the main ingredient in hormone* replacement therapy regimes and can be used to suppress lactation*. In reproductive medicine, oestrogens can be used to treat deficiency or excessive viscosity of the cervical* mucus which may interfere with sperm penetration. Oestrogens can be administered orally, by skin patches, as gels or implants, and vaginally.

Anti-oestrogens such as clomiphene* and tamoxifen* increase endogenous FSH* concentrations by their action on the hypothalamus* and pituitary* and lead to the stimulation of follicular development in anovulatory* patients.

In men, oestrogen concentrations are low. They are derived by conversion from testosterone* by aromatase, found in fatty tissues. Oestrogens are metabolized in the liver and liver failure may cause gynaecomastia*. This can also occur in very obese men and in athletes taking high doses of anabolic* steroids which are aromatized to oestrogens. Oestrogen administration in men lowers the sperm count. Oestrogens can be used to treat advanced prostatic* cancer; this can produce feminizing side effects.

oestrone (E₁): the main postmenopausal* oestrogen* produced by the adrenal* glands and by peripheral conversion of androgens* in fat. This is a weaker oestrogen* than oestradiol*, but it can still stimulate endometrial* proliferation.

oligo-astheno-terato-zoospermia (OAT syndrome): a disturbance involving all three semen variables, i.e. concentration less than 20 million/ml, motility fewer than 50% with forward progression, or less than 25% with rapid progression, and normal morphology less than 30%. These conditions are associated with severely lowered fertility rates, for which no known treatment is available. ICSI* can, however, be used to achieve fertilization of the partner's oocytes*.

oligohydramnios: the presence of less than the normal amount of amniotic* fluid, as assessed clinically and by ultrasound*. It is the opposite of hydramnios* (also known as polyhydramnios). Deficiency of liquor may be associated with abnormalities of the fetal urinary tract as fetal urine is one of the main constituents of the amniotic fluid. A reduced volume of liquor may also reflect poor placental blood flow and thus be associated with retarded fetal growth. Oligohydramnios may cause fetal postural deformities, such as talipes (club foot) and interfere with normal fetal lung development.

oligomenorrhoea: infrequent menstrual periods, i.e. a cycle of between 6 weeks and 6 months. This is common in the early cycles in girls at the menarche* when regular ovulation* is not yet established. In most women, oligomenorrhoea is associated with polycystic* ovarian syndrome and anovulation* and thus subfertility. Some women with oligomenorrhoea ovulate occasionally, but are subfertile as ovulation is infrequent and unpredictable.

In women wishing to conceive, oligomenorrhoea is treated with ovarian* stimulation: clomiphene* citrate is the drug of choice and induces ovulation in more than 70% of patients, but the pregnancy rate is much lower. Women who do not ovulate, or ovulate but do not conceive, after 4 to 6 courses of clomiphene, can be treated with gonadotrophins* for ovarian* stimulation. Surgical treatment with ovarian diathermy may be employed in women with PCO syndrome. Women who do not wish to conceive are best treated with oral contraceptives which induce regular bleeding and protect the endometrium* against hyperplasia*.

oligospermia: a non-specific term meaning subnormal semen* quality.

oligozoospermia: reduced sperm concentration in the semen (less than 20 million/ml according to the WHO* definition). The significance of a low sperm count is debatable since a man's fertility depends more on sperm function, reflected by morphology* and motility, than on sperm numbers. Hormonal treatment is rarely successful because these patients do not usually have identifiable hormone deficiencies.

oncogenes: genes* involved in the conversion of certain host cells into cancer cells. Oncogenes produce proteins* that are involved in the regulation of cell proliferation. As a result, the cancerous cells lack restraints on their division and proliferate out of control.

oocyte: (*syn.* egg, ovum or female gamete*, Fig. 17.) Primary oocytes are formed in the fetal ovary* and persist in primordial follicles* until growth, maturation* and ovulation* occur or until the follicles become atretic*. In fetal life, the two ovaries contain several million primordial follicles. By birth this number has declined to about 2 million and even before puberty*, the majority of oocytes have undergone atresia*.

Oocyte maturation involves completion of meiosis* and expulsion of the first polar* body. A second polar body containing half the chromosome* content is expelled at fertilization*. The mature human oocyte, surrounded by the zona* pellucida, is about 0.15 mm in diameter. Although many follicles with their oocytes are recruited in any one cycle, usually only one follicle becomes dominant and most women, at ovulation, release only one oocyte per cycle. Fertility drugs (see ovarian stimulation) can promote the growth of many follicles, each containing an oocyte. The menopause* occurs when the supply of oocytes is depleted to less than about 1000. (See also follicle, germinal vesicle, maturation, ovulation, egg donation, cryopreservation, micromanipulation.)

oocyte collection: the aspiration of pre-ovulatory oocytes* from their follicles* for use in IVF* or GIFT*. In IVF, collection was originally done by laparoscopic* needle aspiration of follicles; now the transvaginal route with ultrasound* guidance is generally used. Sedation, local anaesthesia or a light general anaesthetic may be used.

Oocyte collection is performed approximately 34 hours after the LH* surge in natural cycles or after the administration of hCG* in stimulated cycles.

oocyte donation: see egg donation.

oogenesis (Fig. 18): the process by which a female organism makes an oocyte*. In humans, primordial germ* cells migrate to the developing fetal ovary. They first multiply by mitosis* to form several million precursor cells known as oogonia*. The oogonia enter meiosis* mainly during the late first and early second trimester* of pregnancy. Meiosis arrests shortly after its

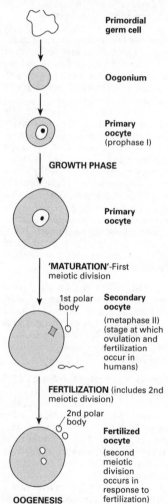

Fig. **18**. Oogenesis. Development of the mature human oocyte. Note that the second meiotic division and expulsion of the second polar body are completed during fertilization, which is shown by the presence of two pronuclei.

initiation, resulting in primary oocytes which become surrounded by ovarian cells to form primordial* follicles, but many developing oocytes become atretic* and are lost before birth. The oocyte pool formed during fetal life is finite.

A small proportion of follicles* initiates growth daily, throughout childhood as well as adulthood, until the menopause*, when the number of oocytes remaining falls below a threshold of about 1000. Ovulation* occurs approximately monthly during the reproductive phase of life, so only about 400 of the many available oocytes are normally ovulated. The vast majority of follicles and their enclosed oocytes succumb.

Maturity is normally attained only by oocytes in pre-ovulatory follicles. In response to the midcycle LH* surge, the primary oocyte reinitiates meiosis, expels the first polar* body and progresses to the second metaphase of meiosis, where it arrests again. At this stage, the mature oocyte is ovulated and is available for fertilization*.

oogonium: diploid* precursor of the oocyte*, formed from primordial germ* cells by repeated mitoses*. Oogonia are formed in the fetal ovary from about 9–10 weeks of gestation. (see oogenesis.)

oolemma (Fig. 17): also known, in humans, as the vitelline membrane: this membrane encloses the oocyte* and is the inner boundary of the perivitelline* space, i.e. the area between the oocyte and the zona* pellucida. The fertilizing sperm binds to the oolemma and penetrates it. Once activated, the oocyte blocks the entry of further spermatozoa by the fusion of its cortical* granules with the oolemma, releasing enzymes* which harden the zona* pellucida. (See zona reaction.)

ooplasm: the cytoplasm* of the oocyte*.

oophorectomy: the surgical removal of one (unilateral) or both (bilateral) ovaries*. This may be carried out for the treatment of benign or malignant ovarian tumours and of uterine cancer. Bilateral oophorectomy is routinely performed by most gynaecologists at the time of hysterectomy* in women who have reached the menopause* to avoid possible later development of ovarian* cancer. In younger women, the ovaries are usually conserved whenever safely possible. Young women, successfully treated for ovarian cancer by bilateral oophorectomy may be offered treatment with donor oocytes (see egg* donation) to achieve a pregnancy,

oophoritis: inflammation of the ovaries: this is usually associated with salpingitis* and pelvic* inflammatory disease.

orchidectomy: removal of a testis*, for example for malignant disease.

orchiometer: device for measuring testicular* size by comparison with a graduated series of ovoids of known volume or length.

orchiopexy (orchidopexy): operation to bring an undescended* or incorrectly situated testis* to its correct position in the scrotum*. If carried out before the age of 5 years (preferably 2 years), later infertility may be prevented.

orchitis: inflammation of the testis*, generally indistinguishable from epididymitis* or epididymo-orchitis*. It is usually caused by a mumps* virus* infection (mumps orchitis), but can also be caused by Coxsackie or herpes* viruses. Testicular damage with infertility and hormone deficiency (hypogonadism*) may follow. Immune orchitis is caused by antisperm* antibodies and may lead to rete* testis obstruction.

orgasm: the intensely pleasurable climax of sexual activity. In the male this is usually associated with ejaculation*. Failure to achieve orgasm (anorgasmia) may be due to insufficient stimulation or psychological factors, or result from central nervous system disorders or the use of certain drugs.

osteoporosis: loss of bone mass which particularly affects the bones of the vertebral column and limbs. Bone mass is the result of a continuous balance between bone formation and bone resorption. Peak bone mass is reached by the age of 30 years and after this there is a slow decline in both sexes. In women this is greatly accelerated by the menopause*. Other conditions such as secondary amenorrhoea* and hypogonadism* in which low oestrogen* concentrations prevail have a similar effect. Osteoporosis is also associated with high concentrations of corticosteroids as seen in Cushing's* syndrome and consumers of anabolic* steroids for body building.

Bone loss leads to deformities from curvature of the vertebral column and loss of height; the brittle nature of the bones causes pain and the tendency to fractures. These occur typically in the spine, hip and lower forearm. Bone mineral density can be measured by X-rays and this can be used to identify patients at risk of rapid bone loss and fractures. Special risk factors, apart from low oestrogen or high corticosteroid concentrations already mentioned, include a thin bodily habitus, positive family history and physical inactivity. The use of bone density measurement as a screening* technique in all postmenopausal women, to determine who would benefit most from hormone* replacement therapy, is controversial.

Hormone* replacement therapy (HRT), if continued for at least 5, possibly 10, years after the onset of the menopause is highly effective in preventing osteoporosis or at least postponing its onset. Treatment of established osteoporosis is difficult and centres on the use of analgesics, vitamin D preparations, biophosphonates and high dosage HRT.

In men, hypogonadism can also lead to osteoporosis.

ovarian cancer: this malignancy arises chiefly from the surface lining of the ovary*, although less commonly tumours arise from the germ* cells themselves or from the substance of the ovary (gonadal stroma).

There is an established relationship between the incidence of ovarian cancer and reproductive performance: pregnancy confers a measure of protection, as does the use of hormonal contraception*. It is speculated that surface 'trauma' from ovulation may have a carcinogenic effect, suppressed by both pregnancy and contraception.

The peak incidence of ovarian cancer around the menopause* further suggests that endogenous gonadotrophin* stimulation may play a role and this may be of concern if extensive use is made of gonadotrophins in infertile patients already at an increased risk of the disorder.

Several epidemiological studies have assessed whether the use of fertility drugs is related to an increased risk of developing ovarian cancer. It has been suggested by some authors that the use of clomiphene* citrate for more than 12 cycles may have a carcinogenic effect, but this has been denied by others. Infertile women are in any case at greater risk and they are also under closer supervision with ultrasound* scans so that tumours in this group of treated women are diagnosed earlier and more frequently. If there is a causal relationship between the use of fertility drugs and the incidence of ovarian cancer, the odds are very small and so far the risk has not been proven.

ovarian failure: failure of the ovary to produce oestradiol* and progesterone* and to achieve oocyte* maturation. This occurs naturally at the menopause*.

Premature* ovarian failure (premature menopause) is ovarian failure before the age of 40 years. It occurs in 1 to 2% of women and may affect very young women in their late teens or twenties; very occasionally it is a transient condition, with spontaneous reversal and return of ovulation*. It may be due to congenital causes (e.g. Turner's* syndrome), auto-immune* disease, pituitary* and nutritional disturbances, other forms of hypogonadism* and Sheehan's* syndrome or it may follow bilateral oophorectomy* or the use of radiotherapy or chemotherapy in young women suffering from malignancies. In some women it represents a natural variation in the number of oocytes present in that individual leading to earlier than usual depletion.

The diagnosis is confirmed by finding a raised serum FSH* concentration and inactive ovaries on ultrasound* scanning. Treatment consists of hormone* replacement therapy to avoid premature bone loss and cardio-vascular disease. Ovulation induction and the use of GnRH* analogues are not appropriate. Those who wish to conceive, require egg* donation which yields a high (40%) pregnancy rate.

ovarian stimulation: the use of fertility drugs to promote the growth of multiple follicles*. Ovarian stimulation without IVF* is used in the management of certain types of amenorrhoea*, hypogonadism* and as adjunct to intra-uterine* insemination.

A variety of regimes exist to achieve ovarian stimulation with clomiphene* citrate and/or gonadotrophins* and these are often preceded by the use of GnRH* analogues to achieve ovarian quiescence before treatment begins. In *in-vitro* fertilization (IVF), the object is to collect several mature oocytes for fertilization as there is a direct relationship between the number of embryos* transferred to the uterus and the incidence of pregnancy.

The most serious complication of ovarian stimulation is the ovarian* hyperstimulation syndrome (OHSS). The occurrence of OHSS is largely controlled by strict monitoring of stimulation treatment by ultrasound* scans and measurements of serum oestradiol* concentrations. The possible carcinogenic effect of ovarian stimulatory drugs is discussed under ovarian* cancer.

ovarian hyperstimulation syndrome (OHSS): the excessive response of the ovaries*, following the production of a large number of follicles* by gonadotrophic* stimulation in ART*. Careful monitoring of ovarian function by serial oestradiol* concentrations and ultrasound* scans is used to detect women at risk of developing OHSS.

Mild OHSS occurs in about 3% of women treated with gonadotrophins and women with the polycystic* ovarian syndrome are particularly susceptible. In mild OHSS, patients experience abdominal heaviness, swelling and discomfort and there is bilateral ovarian enlargement with cysts up to 5 cm in diameter. In moderate OHSS, the ovaries are larger and patients experience more abdominal pain as well as nausea and vomiting. Severe OHSS

occurs in less than 1% of patients. They have massive ovarian enlargement with fluid accumulation in the abdominal and pleural cavities, gross changes in the blood chemistry, a risk of thrombosis* and death. Severe OHSS is a medical emergency and requires hospital admission for intensive treatment; its aetiology is not fully understood.

ovarian wedge resection: surgical excision of part of the ovarian* cortex and stroma, originally employed in the management of the Stein*–Leventhal (polycystic* ovarian) syndrome. Results in terms of restoring normal menstruation* and ovulation* were very good, but infertility persisted in some cases due to the formation of post-operative adhesions*. Whilst this risk can be reduced by the use of microsurgery* or laparoscopic surgery, fertility drugs are now generally used as first line treatment. Recently laparoscopic ovarian diathermy, a much less invasive procedure than wedge resection, has emerged as an effective treatment for PCO patients who do not conceive after 3 to 6 courses of clomiphene* citrate.

ovariotomy: the surgical removal of an ovary containing a tumour.

ovary: the female gonad*. The two ovaries are flat, oval structures; in the adult woman, each is about 3.5 cm long, 2 cm wide and 1.25 cm thick. They are sited one on each side of the uterus, attached by the ovarian ligaments to the upper outer uterine angles, by the infundibulo-pelvic ligaments to the pelvic side walls and by the mesosalpinx* to the lower border of each Fallopian* tube. The outer aspect of the ovary in mature women is pitted and scarred as a result of repeated ovulations* and corpus* albicans formation.

The outer zone of the ovary, covered by a thin layer of germinal* epithelium, is called the cortex and contains the primordial* follicles with their store of oocytes. The inner zone of the ovary is known as the medulla and consists of a connective tissue network (stroma) supporting blood vessels, lymphatics and nerves.

The ovaries produce mature oocytes which are released at ovulation* and also the female sex hormones* (see oestrogens and progesterone) during a woman's reproductive span of life. Ovarian* failure may be the result of genetic, hormonal, environmental or auto-immune factors. The ovaries undergo continuous activity and change and are therefore particularly likely to develop cystic and neoplastic changes. (See follicle, oocyte, ovulation, ovarian cancer, ovarian failure.)

oviduct: see Fallopian* tube.

ovulation: the process during which a Graafian* follicle* ruptures to release a mature oocyte* with its surrounding cumulus* oophorus. This follows a brief rise in the luteinizing* hormone concentration (LH* surge) which precipitates the final changes in the follicular wall, follicular fluid volume and the oocyte which are the necessary precursors to ovulation.

The first meiotic* division is completed at this stage and half the chromosome* complement discarded as the first polar* body. In humans spontaneous ovulation usually occurs 36 to 38 hours after the initiation of the LH surge. The onset of the surge can be determined by measuring LH concentrations in blood and urine, and the timing of follicular rupture by serial ultrasound* scans. These may be used for the correct timing of artificial* insemination or the transfer of previously frozen embryos.

In assisted* reproductive technology, the administration of hCG* is used to trigger ovulation and time oocyte* collection, particularly if spontaneous LH surges are suppressed by GnRH* analogues. Ovulation in humans usually occurs 14 days before the next expected menstruation, i.e. around day 14 in a 28 day cycle. In longer cycles ovulation occurs later, i.e. around day 19 in a 33 day cycle. Ovulation may be associated with temporary discomfort or pain (see Mittelschmerz) and soon after its occurrence there is a rise in the basal* body temperature due to progesterone* production.

ovum: see oocyte.

ovum pick-up mechanism: the way in which the oocyte* reaches the ampulla* of the Fallopian tube where fertilization* can take place. At ovulation*, the (immobile) oocyte, with its surrounding 'sticky' cumulus* cells, emerges from the ruptured follicle*. Contractions of the tubal fimbriae* enable them to sweep over the ovarian surface to pick up the ovum–cumulus complex which, by a combination of peristalsis and currents set up by the cilia*, is propelled into the tubal ampulla.

Pelvic inflammation* can cause adhesions* involving the fimbriae and mesosalpinx*, destruction of cilia and fibrosis of the tubal musculature and, depending on the severity, lead to subfertility or infertility.

ovum donation: see egg donation.

oxygen free radicals: see free radicals.

P

Pap smear: named after Dr Papanicolaou. See cervical smear.

papaverine: a drug which relaxes smooth muscle, used as a test and treatment for erectile impotence*. If the mechnism of erection* is normal, papaverine usually induces a full erection when injected directly into the erectile tissues of the penis*. Papaverine can cause prolonged erections (priapism) and occasionally scarring of the erectile tissues; for long term treatment, it has largely been replaced by prostaglandin* injections.

papilloma virus: see human papilloma virus.

paracentesis: the removal of accumulated fluid from an enclosed cavity by tapping through a hollow needle, catheter or cannula. The term is usually used to refer to the tapping of ascites* from the peritoneal cavity. This may be for diagnostic purposes (e.g. for bacteriological culture or cytological examination for malignant cells), relief of discomfort from excessive abdominal distension or treatment, e.g. the installation of cytotoxic drugs in advanced cancer. In severe ovarian* hyperstimulation syndrome, massive ascites may sometimes be an indication for paracentesis.

paraplegia: loss of motor and sensory function of both legs, usually due to spinal cord injury (SCI). There may be associated bladder and bowel incontinence and, in men, usually erectile impotence* and ejaculatory* failure. Sperm production and function are usually normal. Semen* may be obtained by penile* vibratory stimulation, rectal electro-ejaculation* or vas* deferens aspiration and can be used for AIH* or IVF* with good prospects of pregnancy.

parity: the number of times a woman has given birth: for example a woman who has never given birth is a 'nullipara'; whilst one who has had at least one child is a multipara. If she has had, for example, 3 children she may be referred to as a 'para 3'. (See also gravidity.)

parthenogenesis: the activation* of an oocyte*, without fertilization* by a spermatozoon*. This occurs in about 1% of oocytes cultured *in vitro*, and the incidence increases with *in vitro* ageing of oocytes. Parthenogenetic activation can be induced by a variety of stimuli (see activation). Parthenogenetic oocytes may enter syngamy* and appear identical to normally fertilized embryos during early cleavage*, but in humans they develop no further because paternally imprinted chromosomes* are absent. (See imprinting.)

partial zona dissection (PZD): see assisted fertilization.

passive immunization: the administration to a patient of human polyclonal antibody* against a specific antigen*. The biggest, and most successful, project in the UK has been the passive immunization programme to reduce the incidence of haemolytic* disease of the newborn. For this, intramuscular anti-Rh(D) antibody (made by immunizing volunteer men) is given to Rh(D) negative women who have no anti-D themselves and have recently given birth to Rh(D) positive infants. The antibody attaches to any Rh(D) positive fetal red blood cells which have entered the maternal circulation during childbirth, and destroys them before the mother becomes immunized. This ensures she does not produce anti-D which could affect future pregnancies.

The standard dose of anti-D is 500 iu. The infant's blood group is checked after delivery and, if the infant is Rh(D) positive, a Kleihauer test is performed on the mother to ensure that the standard dose of anti-D is sufficient, or that further doses are given as appropriate. The anti-D is administered to the mother as soon as possible and no later than 48 hours after delivery. Anti-D is also given to all Rh(D) negative women after a miscarriage* or pregnancy termination. If the partner is himself Rh(D) negative, such treatment is not needed and not given. (See also haemolytic disease of the newborn.)

pelvic inflammatory disease (PID): this term includes endometritis*, salpingitis*, salpingo-oophoritis*, tubo-ovarian abscess* and pelvic peritonitis. Whilst infections may follow delivery, miscarriage*, termination of pregnancy, tuberculosis* of the genital tract, or intra-abdominal conditions such as perforated appendicitis*, the term PID is generally applied to conditions resulting from sexually* transmitted diseases. The peak incidence is in young sexually active women and pre-disposing factors include frequent or recent change of sexual partner, failure to use barrier methods of contraception*, and use of an intra-uterine* contraceptive device (IUCD).

Infection spreads from the lower genital tract; *Chlamydia* *trachomatis* and *Neisseria* *gonorrhoea* are the commonest infecting organisms. In acute cases there is a raised temperature, lower abdominal pain, vaginal discharge and pain on intercourse (dyspareunia*), but in many cases (particularly of chlamydial origin) there is little or no pain so that diagnosis is difficult and often the patient is unaware of the infection.

Early treatment with appropriate antibiotics is effective, but if delayed or inadequate, chronic pelvic pain, extra-uterine* pregnancy and tubal infertility may follow. Re-infection from untreated, and frequently symptomless, sexual partners leads to repeated episodes of PID. The risk of extra-uterine pregnancy and infertility is directly related to the number of episodes of infection a woman has suffered. Sex education of young people, contact* tracing and epidemiological surveillance as well as prompt diagnosis and treatment are necessary to combat this major cause of infertility. (See also epididymitis.)

penile prosthesis: a semi-rigid or inflatable device, surgically implanted into the penis* in cases of irreversible organic impotence*, for example those resulting from spinal injury.

penile vibrator: a vibratory stimulator applied to the penis* which induces ejaculation* in about 50% of paraplegic* men. Semen* thus obtained is used for AIH*.

penis (Fig. 15): the organ of copulation according to which male gender* is assigned to the newborn. Both urine and semen are discharged through the urethra* which traverses the penis. Due to the presence of three longitudinal bodies of spongy erectile tissue, the normally flaccid organ can stiffen in response to sexual stimulation so that penetrative intercourse can be achieved. (See also erection, ejaculation, impotence.)

pentoxifylline (oxpentifylline): a drug, similar to caffeine, which improves sperm function *in vitro* by stimulating motility; it acts as an anti-oxidant by scavenging free radicals (see reactive oxygen species) which occur in the semen* of most infertile men and adversely affect sperm motility and fertilizing ability. Although pentoxifylline has been shown to improve fertilization* and embryo* transfer rates in some IVF* studies, pregnancy rates were not increased. Claims for its efficacy by oral administration to subfertile males have not been substantiated. Its use has largely been superseded by ICSI*.

percutaneous epididymal sperm aspiration (PESA): see epididymal sperm aspiration, surgical sperm retrieval.

Pergonal: a proprietary brand of human* menopausal gonadotrophin (hMG) widely used in the treatment of anovulatory* infertility and hypogonadotrophic* hypogonadism, and for ovarian* stimulation in assisted* reproductive technology. Pergonal is supplied in powder form in 1 ml ampoules, each containing 75 iu FSH* and 75 iu LH*. It is derived from the urine of post-menopausal women (see hMG). (See also recombinant human FSH.)

perineum (Fig. 27): the area between the vaginal* orifice and the anus which covers the muscular perineal body. An episiotomy is an incision made in the perineum in the second stage of labour to facilitate delivery and avoid perineal laceration.

peritoneal oocyte sperm transfer (POST): transfer of a number of oocytes* (usually one to three), retrieved by follicular aspiration (see oocyte collection) and mixed with a sample of prepared* semen, into the pouch* of Douglas. The route for the transfer is by needle puncture of the vaginal* vault. Occasional pregnancies have been achieved in couples with unexplained* infertility, but the technique is now considered unsatisfactory and is seldom practized.

peritoneoscopy: see laparoscopy.

peritoneum: the thin serous membrane which lines the abdominal cavity and surrounds the organs within it. It has a smooth surface which enables the abdominal organs to move in relation to each other. The peritoneum which lines the abdominal and pelvic walls is known as the parietal peritoneum, whereas the visceral peritoneum coats the outer surface of the abdominal organs.

The pelvic peritoneal cavity is a subdivision of the general peritoneal cavity. In women, the ovaries are the only intra-abdominal organs that are not covered by visceral peritoneum and the abdominal* ostium of the Fallopian* tube provides the only communication between the peritoneal cavity and the lower genital tract through the lumen of the tubes and uterus; this continuity of the peritoneal cavity with the lower genital tract can be a particularly dangerous pathway for ascending infection. The peritoneum is very sensitive to inflammation (peritonitis) and readily develops adhesions* in response to the inflammatory process. Peritonitis may arise from ascending pelvic infections, perforated appendicitis, injury or disease of the bowel, or tuberculosis. (See also pelvic inflammatory disease.)

perivitelline space (Fig. 17): the area between the inner surface of the zona* pellucida and the oolemma* (which is also known as the vitelline membrane).

The polar* bodies are released from the oocyte* into the perivitelline space, as are the contents of the cortical* granules in the zona* reaction. (See also cortical granules, oolemmma.)

Peyronie's disease: a local condition affecting the erectile bodies of the penis*, common in diabetics*. A small mass within the penis, associated with transient impotence*, resolves over a period of 12 to 18 months, usually resulting in a curve or deviation of the erection, which is otherwise firm. In rare cases, the deviation prevents penetrative intercourse and operative correction or a penile implant are indicated.

Pfannenstiel incision: a transverse incision of the abdominal cavity just above the pubic symphysis, widely used in gynaecological surgery and for Caesarean section. Whilst this is sometimes called the 'bikini' incision, it is employed not merely for cosmetic purposes, but because it heals better, with less likelihood of incisional hernia, than a vertical approach to the pelvic cavity and its organs.

phantom pregnancy: see pseudocyesis.

phenotype: the physical appearance of an organism; the result of both the genotype* of the organism and the effects of the environment in which it has existed. For example, a full description of the phenotype of a person with Down's* syndrome would include an account of their visible physical characteristics, their internal anatomy and physiology and their mental (including emotional) state.

phenylketonuria: a hereditary disease caused by a recessive* allele*: the liver fails to produce the enzyme* phenylalanine hydroxylase, so that phenylalanine accumulates in the circulation. This causes severe damage to the brain of the newborn. Affected babies are put on a diet low in phenylalanine from birth. The disease occurs in about 1 in 10 000 births. In the UK all babies are screened* (by a heel prick to obtain blood, the Guthrie test) at birth. Prenatal* diagnosis is available for women identified by having had a previous affected baby.

phimosis: tightening of the opening of the foreskin of the penis*, so that it cannot be retracted. This is a normal phenomenon in many newborn babies, but, if it persists, circumcision is necessary, especially if there are recurrent infections or the flow of urine is restricted. (See also prepuce.)

Phimosis is also the term applied to a narrowing down to a pin-point opening of the abdominal ostium* of the Fallopian* tube. This is the aftermath of inflammation* and causes inversion of the fimbriae* with consequent impairment of the ovum* pick-up mechanism.

pinopodes: apical protrusions which appear on the endometrial* surface in the luteal* phase of the menstrual* cycle and may be involved in the ability of the uterus* to accept an implanting* embryo.

pituitary gland (*syn.* hypophysis): this small endocrine* gland (weighing about 5 g) is sited in the pituitary fossa at the base of the skull and is attached to the forebrain by a stalk. The anterior lobe of the gland contains acidophil cells which produce prolactin* and growth* hormone and basophil cells which produce thyroid* stimulating hormone (TSH), follicle* stimulating hormone (FSH), luteinizing* hormone (LH) and adrenal* cortical stimulating hormone (ACTH). These hormones (with the exception of prolactin) are produced in a pulsatile manner in response to releasing hormones (e.g. GnRH*) produced in the hypothalamus* and are transported in the hypothalamic–pituitary portal venous system (Fig. 12). Complex feedback mechanisms exist to modify anterior pituitary hormone production, e.g. oestrogens* exert both a negative and a positive feedback on LH production at different stages of the menstrual* cycle.

In women, failure of the anterior pituitary to produce sufficient FSH and LH causes hypogonadotrophic* hypogonadism with low oestrogen* concentrations, amenorrhoea* and anovulation*. In men, pituitary insufficiency is a rare cause of infertility and is associated with low testosterone* concentrations and hypogonadism*.

Gonadotrophin* treatment is effective in both sexes. If there is generalized impairment of anterior pituitary hormone production, panhypopituitarism results (see postpartum pituitary necrosis, Sheehan's syndrome). If pituitary failure occurs in childhood, infantilism and failure of growth occur.

The posterior lobe of the pituitary gland is effectively a neural extension of the hypothalamus*. Hypothalamic cells produce vasopressin (anti-diuretic hormone) and oxytocin (which stimulates uterine contractions); these are carried down neuronal axons as granules and are stored in the terminals in the pituitary gland until released.

pituitary adenoma (*syn.* prolactinoma): a benign overgrowth of pituitary cells leading to raised serum prolactin* concentrations. An adenoma may be less than 10 mm in size, when it is called a microadenoma. Clinically, in women, amenorrhoea* and galactorrhoea* occur, whilst in men there may be impotence*. Diagnosis is usually made by CT and MRI scans and treatment is with long-term dopamine* agonists (bromocriptine* or cabergoline) which are highly effective in restoring fertility. Surgical treatment (trans-sphenoidal excision) is occasionally required for large tumours, which may cause pressure on the optic chiasma with resultant loss of peripheral vision.

placebo: a pharmacologically inactive substance. Placebos are administered to patients taking part in drug trials*. After informed consent, patients are randomly chosen for treatment by either drug or placebo and the outcome in the two groups is assessed. In a cross-over trial, a group of patients may be treated first with drug, then with placebo, and compared with a group treated first with placebo, then with drug.

Several days of placebo (i.e. inactive) tablets are included in certain oral contraceptive* and hormone* replacement packs and withdrawal bleeds occur during these days.

Placebos may also be given to patients to attempt to provide relief from psychosomatic illness.

placenta: the more or less round, flat, spongy organ, entirely fetal in origin, formed from the primitive trophectoderm* at the site of implantation* of the blastocyst*.

The placenta transfers nutrients and oxygen from the maternal to the fetal circulation and waste products and carbon dioxide in the opposite direction. Hormones*, antibodies*, many drugs*, viruses* and some bacteria* can cross the placental barrier. The placenta itself produces many hormones, including hCG (see human chorionic gonadotrophin), essential for the continuation of the pregnancy, oestriol*, progesterone* and prolactin*.

Inadequate bloodflow from the maternal circulation to the placental site may result in low birth weight babies. Binovular* twins have two separate placentas, though there may be some apparent fusion; uniovular twins usually share one placenta. The placenta is expelled in the third stage of labour, after delivery of the baby. Retention of parts of the placenta in the uterus may cause post-partum haemorrhage or infection.

placental proteins: large molecular weight proteins* produced by the placenta* and detectable in maternal serum; the function of many of them remains unknown. Human* chorionic gonadotrophin (hCG) can be detected soon after implantation* and assays of it form the basis of modern pregnancy* tests. Serial asessment of hCG and human placental lactogen have been used in the past in an attempt to predict fetal well-being, both in threatened miscarriage* and in growth retardation. Ultrasound* scanning and Doppler* assessments have in general replaced their use. HCG measurements are included in the maternal serum screening for Down's* syndrome.

pneumoperitoneum: instillation of gas to distend the peritoneal cavity as a necessary preliminary to laparoscopy*. For diagnostic and operative laparoscopy, 100% carbon dioxide is used, but for laparoscopic oocyte* collection for IVF*, a mixture of 5% carbon dioxide, 5% oxygen and 90% nitrogen is used.

polar body (Fig. 17): a small membrane-bound cellular structure emitted from an oocyte*, consisting of nuclear material* and a small amount of cytoplasm*.

The first polar body is released at the end of the first meiotic* division. It contains half the recombined* genetic material of the oocyte* but only a tiny fraction of the cytoplasm. The second polar body is released as the oocyte completes the second meiotic division, normally in response to penetration by the fertilizing spermatozoon*; it appears similar to the first, but contains a haploid* chromosome complement.

The polar bodies have no known further role: they are not viable cells due to their lack of cytoplasm and eventually degenerate. The extrusion of the polar bodies allows the developing oocyte to retain almost all of the cytoplasm, whilst reducing the chromosome complement from 46 to 23. (See meiosis.)

polycystic ovaries (Fig. 19): a common finding on ultrasound* scanning of the ovaries*, characterized by the peripheral distribution of ten or more small follicles* in the ovarian cortex, with a thickened central stroma (the hormonally inactive connective tissue component of the ovary). The presence of polycystic ovaries may be an incidental finding and is not necessarily associated with any particular clinical abnormalities. Polycystic ovaries are thought to be inherited in a non-Mendelian fashion and are linked with premature balding in men.

polycystic ovarian syndrome (PCOS): this is the commonest cause of ovarian dysfunction in women in the reproductive phase of life and consists of the presence of polycystic* ovaries on ultrasound* scanning together with various symptoms and signs. There is a widespread spectrum of manifestations of the condition, but hyperandrogenism* is the main feature. The serum LH* concentration is usually raised above 10 iu/L and the serum testosterone concentration may also be elevated.

In the mildest form of PCOS, affected women may have no menstrual irregularity and ovulate normally, but may take longer than average to conceive* and have a higher risk of

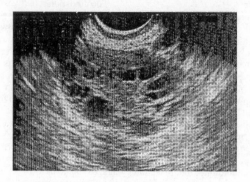

Fig. **19**. Polycystic ovaries. Ultrasound scan showing the typical peripheral distribution of multiple microcysts in the ovarian cortex.

spontaneous miscarriage*. More often, there are menstrual irregularities such as oligomenorrhoea* or secondary amenorrhoea* and thus failure of ovulation*. Hirsutism*, acne, seborrhoea and obesity* are common but not obligatory for the diagnosis. The most severe degree of PCOS is the Stein*–Leventhal syndrome with obesity, hirsutism, amenorrhoea and infertility.

Recently PCOS has been linked with hyperinsulinism and an increased risk of cardiovascular disease. There is no increased incidence of ovarian* cancer, but a very small risk of uterine (endometrial*) cancer in untreated women.

Treatment is symptomatic. In women who do not wish to conceive, a low dose oral contraceptive* pill may be recommended to induce regular cyclical bleeding. In those with hirsutism or acne, cyproterone* acetate and oestrogens* may be used. Those wishing to conceive may be treated in the first place with clomiphene* citrate in doses of 50 to 100 mg/day for 5 days at monthly intervals. This is effective in restoring normal menstruation with ovulation* in 75% of cases, but pregnancy rates are only 30% and there is a high incidence of spontaneous miscarriage*. If conception has not occurred after 6 months treatment with clomiphene, gonadotrophins* (see human menopausal gonadotrophin) may be used with caution, as these patients are very susceptible to developing the ovarian* hyperstimulation syndrome. Down regulation with GnRH* analogues (see gonadotrophin releasing hormone, also Buserelin) has been used in an attempt to lower the raised LH concentration and reduce the risk of miscarriage.

Originally the Stein–Leventhal syndrome was treated by a surgical ovarian* wedge resection. Properly performed this had a very high success rate, even in patients with a less severe clinical picture, but its indiscriminate use without proper microsurgical* technique led to a high incidence of pelvic adhesions* and the operation fell into disrepute. More recently, laparoscopic* wedge resection, ovarian diathermy and laser* vaporization have been introduced as an effective form of treatment and alternative to hormonal ovarian stimulation.

polymenorrhoea: cyclical menstruation, normal in amount, at shorter than average intervals, e.g. every 21 days. Ovulation* may occur regularly, in which case it is the follicular* phase of the cycle which is short. If there is anovulation, treatment with clomiphene* citrate or gonado-trophins* is required for conception.

polymerase chain reaction (PCR): a technique used in genetic* diagnosis. It was initially used to isolate and amplify a gene sequence several milli-onfold, so that it could be analysed. The method relies upon repeated cycles of denaturation of DNA* into sin-gle strands; attachment (annealing) of small primers of DNA with sequences complementary to areas just outside the sequence of interest; and extension of the primers through the sequence using an enzyme specific for this function and which is not inactivated by the high temperatures needed for denaturation. The newly formed DNA can then act as a template for more cycles of ampli-fication.

In this way, particular genes, or important fragments of genes, can be amplified from as little as a single copy to many million copies in a few hours. A similar technique can be used to am-plify RNA*. This important technique has revolutionized the analysis of very small quantities of material, such as oocytes*, spermatozoa* and embryos*, or single cell biopsies*, and can be used in preimplantation* diagnosis of genetic* disorders.

polyp: an adenoma* (benign growth) arising on a stalk from mucous mem-branes. This is a very common condi-tion and polyps are found in the nose, sinuses and bowel. In the female geni-tal tract, they frequently arise from the endocervical epithelium* and protrude from the external os of the cervix*, sometimes causing discharge or inter-menstrual bleeding. Polyps also often arise from the endometrium*, when they may cause heavy menstruation or intermenstrual bleeding.

polyploidy: the condition when a cell* has a multiple of the normal comple-ment of chromosomes*. In humans, virtually all cells (except for the gam-etes*) are diploid* and contain 46 chromosomes. The commonest form of polyploidy is triploidy* when the cell contains three times the normal hapl-oid* complement. Polyploidy results from faulty meiosis* or fertilization* (see polyspermy) and, being incompat-ible with normal development, nearly always leads to early miscarriage* (see anembryonic pregnancy).

In human IVF*, polyploid embryos can occur because of abnormal fertili-zation, for example triploidy from the fertilization of an oocyte* by two sper-matozoa*. Such abnormal embryos are not transferred to the uterus, although they may develop *in vitro* as far as the blastocyst* stage.

polyspermy: the condition when an oocyte* is penetrated by more than one spermatozoon*. Triploid* or tetraploid (see polyploidy) embryos may result. Polyspermic embryos can be identi-fied *in vitro* by the presence of more than two pronuclei*. Their transfer is avoided in *in* * *vitro* fertilization* treat-ment because of the risk of producing a polyploid pregnancy or hydatidiform* mole. (See triploidy, zona reaction.)

Pomeroy operation: a form of female sterilization*, consisting of the exci-sion of a loop of the isthmus of each Fallopian* tube. The operation has largely been superseded by laparo-scopic* sterilization techniques, but is sometimes still used when sterilization is performed at the time of another ab-dominal operations such as Caesarean* section.

postcoital test (PCT): this is a sim-ple, cheap and basic infertility in-vestigation. It assesses the quality of the cervical* mucus and the presence and viability of spermatozoa*. Sper-matozoa require an adequate amount of clear, fluid (oestrogenic) mucus as safe haven from the acidity of the vagina and for migration to the upper female genital tract.

The test is performed just before the estimated date of ovulation*, some 6 to 12 hours after normal, unprotected intercourse. Some advise sexual absti-nence for the male for 2–3 days before the test, but the need for this is ques-tionable. After passage of a speculum*, a small amount of cervical* mucus is aspirated and immediately examined microscopically.

The commonest cause of a poor cervical mucus is inappropriate tim-ing of the test: performed too early, it may not be fully oestrogenic; per-formed too late, it may have become highly viscous under the influence of progesterone*. A gross deficiency of mucus (dry cervix) may result from amputation of the cervix and certain other operations which destroy cervical glands. The presence of many white blood cells may indicate inflammatory conditions, prejudicial to conception*.

An estimate is made of the number and activity of spermatozoa observed microscopically. This may vary from hundreds to none. The test is considered adequate if 5 to 10 freely mobile spermatozoa are seen per high power field. Their motility is assessed: it may vary from highly active progressive movement to sluggish, or no, motility. Clumping, shaking or agglutination (head to head or tail to tail) may suggest the presence of antisperm* antibodies.

An unsatisfactory PCT is due to incorrect timing, poor cervical mucus, poor semen or inadequate coitus and indicates the need for further investigations. A good PCT indicates that intercourse is adequate (no vaginismus* or premature ejaculation*), that the male is likely to be fertile and that the woman is normal up to the level of the cervix. The prognosis for conception is good in the presence of a good PCT, providing ovulation occurs and the Fallopian* tubes are healthy. A single unsatisfactory test is of little significance and so the test may have to be repeated. Gynaecologists are aware of the stress experienced by some couples through having to perform coitus to order.

postpartum pituitary necrosis (Sheehan's syndrome): this is a rare consequence of severe bloodloss, vascular shock and lowering of blood* pressure due to haemorrhage at the time of delivery. Bloodflow through the pituitary*–hypothalamic* circulation is reduced, resulting in thrombosis* and necrosis of the pituitary gland with loss of its function. Patients exhibit hypogonadotrophic* hypogonadism (first sign: no return of menstruation after delivery), as well as evidence of thyroid* and adrenal* cortex impairment. Replacement of deficient hormones is required.

Potter's syndrome: a congenital abnormality with absence, or severe dysfunction, of the kidneys as the chief feature. Due to lack of urine secretion by the fetus, there is oligohydramnios* and failure of fetal lung development. Affected babies die soon after birth.

pouch of Douglas (*syn.* recto-vaginal pouch): the lowermost extension of the peritoneal cavity, situated between the uterus* and cervix* in front and rectum behind. The ovaries* and Fallopian* tubes are usually present in the pouch, together with some peritoneal fluid. The pouch is palpated during vaginal examination through the posterior fornix*; blood (from an extra*-uterine pregnancy) or pus (from a pelvic abscess) can be aspirated or drained from the pouch through the vagina*. In assisted* reproductive technology, the pouch of Douglas can be used as a route for transvaginal oocyte* collection and also for peritoneal* oocyte and sperm transfer (POST).

pre-antral follicle: ovarian follicle* which has begun to grow, but is still a solid mass of cells and does not yet contain follicular* fluid. In humans such follicles are usually less than 0.5 mm in diameter. (See also antrum.)

precocious puberty: in girls this is the onset of breast development before the age of 8 and menstruation* before 10 years. The majority of cases are constitutional (i.e. not associated with any disease) or due to lesions in the central nervous system (congenital abnormalities, hypothalamic* tumours or following encephalitis). Hypothyroidism* and tumours of the ovaries* or adrenals* are rare causes. Premature epiphyseal closure, if untreated, can lead to short stature. Treatment is with GnRH* analogues, cyproterone* acetate, medroxyprogesterone (see depot provera) or Danazol*. Psychological support is important and the long term outlook is excellent.

In boys, precocious puberty, characterized by early virilization*, is very rare and may be due to congenital adrenal hyperplasia (see adrenogenital syndrome) or a testicular Leydig* cell tumour.

prednisolone: a steroid* drug sometimes used to suppress antisperm* antibodies in men. Because treatment may need to be prolonged and may have significant side effects, prednisolone therapy is now rarely used and either IVF* or ICSI* are preferred.

pre-eclampsia (PE): also known as pre-eclamptic toxaemia (PET) or proteinuric pregnancy-induced hypertension, this is the commonest serious complication of pregnancy. Affected women have raised blood* pressure, protein (albumin) in the urine, raised serum urate concentration and usually fluid retention, leading to oedema. The condition presents in the second or third trimester* of pregnancy; it is seen more frequently in women having their first pregnancy under the age of 20 or over 35 years, those with pre-existing hypertension* and those who have multiple* pregnancies. If untreated, eclampsia* can occur, with a risk of maternal death.

Treatment is by control of blood presure and planned, early delivery. Magnesium sulphate is used in severe cases to prevent eclampsia. The use of low dosage aspirin to prevent or delay the onset of PE is under investigation. The condition always resolves after delivery and recurrence in subsequent pregnancies, fathered by the same partner, is rare. The fetus is at risk of prematurity*, growth retardation and, in severe cases, perinatal death. (See mortality rates.)

pregnancy: the state of being gravid, which in humans lasts about 38 weeks and during which a woman is carrying within her an unborn but implanted embryo* or fetus* with its placenta* and membranes (see amnion, chorion: Fig. 20). A woman having her first pregnancy is called a primigravida; if it is her second (or subsequent) pregnancy, she is referred to as a multipara.

Most human pregnancies are singletons, but multiple* pregnancy occurs in about 1 in 80 deliveries (see multiple pregnancy). The commonest abnormality of pregnancy in the first trimester* is miscarriage*; biochemical* pregnancies are another important cause of early* pregnancy loss. Extrauterine* pregnancies are a major health hazard; heterotopic* pregnancies occur more frequently after IVF*.

Pregnancy is diagnosed by a history of amenorrhoea*, clinical examination and specific pregnancy* tests. Antenatal care is provided to monitor the progress of pregnancy and development of the fetus. Prenatal* diagnosis of certain fetal abnormalities can be undertaken. Termination of pregnancy is permissible under certain conditions defined in the Abortion Act (1967). (See also pregnancy reduction, surrogate pregnancy.)

pregnancy rates: the percentage of pregnancies occurring after a given procedure. After assisted* reproductive technology procedures, pregnancy rates are commonly published, but

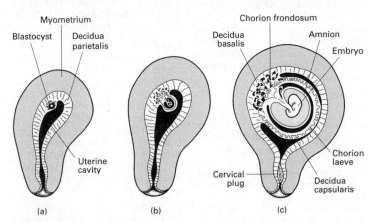

Fig. **20.** Pregnant uterus. Diagram showing the relationship of the embryo and its membranes, the chorion and amnion, to the uterine decidua and cavity during early development. A: three weeks. B: five weeks. C: ten weeks after the last menstruation.

comparison of the results achieved in different clinics is fruitless since the rates depend on a large number of factors which vary from clinic to clinic, viz. different populations or age groups treated, the causes of infertility, different ovarian* stimulation protocols employed and the number of embryos transferred. (See live birth rates.)

pregnancy reduction: procedure by which a high order multiple* pregnancy (i.e. three or more fetuses), which may result from ovarian* stimulation with gonadotrophins*, is reduced to normally a twin or triplet pregnancy. It can also be performed in twin pregnancies if one fetus is found, on antenatal testing, to have a significant congenital abnormality. The operation may be performed by an intracardiac injection of potassium chloride. There is a small risk of miscarriage or intra-uterine growth retardation of the remaining fetus(es). Pregnancy reduction can only be performed in the UK under the terms of the Abortion Act (1967). (See also multiple pregnancy.)

pregnancy tests: old fashioned pregnancy tests (Ascheim*–Zondek, *xenopus*, etc.) have been superseded by the assessment of the presence of the subunit of β hCG* in the blood or urine of a woman. Rapid kit pregnancy tests are colour sensitive with yes/no indicators. These tests can be performed on or after the first day of a missed period with a low false positive rate. Quantitative asessment of hCG may be used to monitor changes in concentrations over time, reflecting for example viability of placental tissue after treatment of an extra-uterine* pregnancy or hydatidiform* mole.

pregnancy toxaemia: see pre-eclampsia.

pre-implantation diagnosis: techniques by which embryos* fertilized *in vitro* are tested for specific genetic* disorders (e.g. cystic* fibrosis), or other characteristics such as sex (in cases of sex*-linked disorders), before transfer into the uterus. Transfer of an affected embryo is thus avoided, as is the need to terminate a pregnancy if a major defect is discovered as a result of later ante-natal* testing (see prenatal diagnosis).

The technique normally involves removing one or two cells (blastomeres*) during late cleavage*. A biopsy* can also be taken from the blastocyst* where more cells are available for removal, potentially improving the reliability of the diagnosis. Some analyses may also be performed on first and/or second polar* bodies, removed from the unfertilized or recently fertilized oocyte. Removal of cells at such early stages of development does not prejudice subsequent normal development of the embryo. Biopsied cells are analysed, using either polymerase* chain reaction (PCR) or fluorescence* *in situ* hybridization (FISH). Rapid amplification of genetic material by these techniques enables analyses to be concluded in a matter of hours, thus allowing unaffected embryos to be transferred in time for implantation*.

Analyses employing PCR and FISH can be used to diagnose fetal sex, chromosome* disorders such as aneuploidy* and specific gene* defects. Cystic* fibrosis, Duchenne* muscular dystrophy, Lesch–Nyhan* syndrome, Tay–Sachs* disease and some of the haemoglobinopathies* have been successfully diagnosed. In the UK, the diagnosis of embryonic sex is permitted only in order to avoid sex-linked* disorders.

premature ovarian failure (POF): the occurrence of the menopause* before the age of 40; this affects between 1 and 2% of women. See ovarian failure.

prematurity: delivery before the 37th completed week, calculated from the beginning of the last menstrual period. Severe prematurity is associated with respiratory problems for the fetus. These may be prevented by the administration of steroids* to women in labour before the 34th week. Problems with fluid balance, jaundice, infection, intraventricular haemorrhage, hypoglycaemia and heat loss can also lead to handicap or death. (See mortality rates, perinatal mortality.)

premenstrual tension (PMT): symptoms occurring during the late luteal* phase of the menstrual cycle; these are thought to be related to changing concentrations of ovarian hormones*, particularly progesterone*, in women with ovulatory* cycles.

The symptoms may include irritability, tearfulness, aggression, lack of concentration, bloatedness, headaches, clumsiness and breast discomfort. A detailed symptom chart needs to be assessed to confirm at least one symptom-free week postmenstrually. General support, with advice on diet and exercise, is beneficial. Medical treatment is either by suppression of ovulation* by the use of the oral contraceptive* pill, GnRH* analogues or high dose oestrogen* implants, or with vitamin B6, Evening Primrose oil or antidepressants. A high placebo* effect has been reported in many studies. PMT-like symptoms may also be experienced during the progestogenic* phase in women taking cyclical hormone* replacement therapy.

prenatal diagnosis (also antenatal diagnosis): antenatal tests for fetal abnormalities are performed in the first or second trimesters* of pregnancy (as opposed to pre-implantation* diagnosis when the tests are carried out before implantation, necessitating *in vitro* fertilization to generate embryos).

Prenatal tests can be used for screening* (e.g. for neural* tube defects, Down's* syndrome in older women) or for the detection of specific genetic* defects in patients with a previous affected child or a positive family history.

Ultrasound is the simplest, non-invasive technique for detecting anatomical abnormalities of the fetus; tests on specific hormones* and chemical constituents of the mother's blood in pregnancy can also give a risk assessment for Down's syndrome and other chromosomal* abnormalities.

Amniocentesis* and chorionic* villus sampling (CVS) are invasive tests; they allow the establishment of the fetal karyotype* for the exclusion of chromosomal* disorders, the rapid diagnosis of fetal sex and the detection of specific genetic disorders if required. Both methods take 2 to 3 weeks to grow fetal cells in culture to prepare a karyotype. Amniocentesis has fewer complications if performed in the second trimester, but this may necessitate a late termination in the case of an affected fetus; CVS is performed in the first trimester, but has a slightly higher incidence of miscarriage* and has been implicated in the causation of fetal limb deformities. Fetal blood sampling can be performed to detect thalassaemia* and sickle* cell anaemia; this is a highly sophisticated test performed only in specialized centres. (See also amniocentesis, chorionic villus sampling.)

prepared semen: see sperm preparation.

prepuce (foreskin): the skin covering the tip of the penis*. Accumulated secretions under the prepuce are known as smegma. Circumcision is the surgical excision of the prepuce and is performed for religious, social or medical reasons, including phimosis*.

primordial follicle: the smallest type of ovarian follicle*, consisting of a single layer of flattened pre-granulosa cells, surrounding the oocyte*. Primordial follicles are formed in the fetus from about the 18th week of pregnancy and remain in this state until they either begin to grow or undergo atresia* without further development. (See also follicle.)

primordial germ cell: see germ cell.

progesterone: one of the female hormones* produced by the cells of the corpus* luteum under the influence of the pituitary gonadotrophins*. Progesterone controls the luteal* (secretory) phase of the menstrual* cycle, but is only active on tissues primed by oestrogens*. Its main functions are to transform the endometrium* from its proliferative to its secretory state, assist in implantation*, block the ascent of further spermatozoa* by increasing the viscosity of the cervical* mucus and prevent the onset of menstruation to ensure the safety of the early pregnancy.

For diagnostic purposes, progestogens* may be given for about 7 days to women complaining of oligomenorrhoea* or amenorrhoea* to induce a withdrawal bleed; this will only occur in women whose endometrium* has been primed with endogenous oestrogens*. In assisted reproduction procedures, progesterone may be administered in tablet form, by intramuscular injection or in vaginal pessaries for luteal* phase support after embryo* transfer. Progestogens* may also be used in the treatment of menorrhagia* or endometriosis*. Used in the new intra-uterine* contraceptive devices, they provide an excellent form of contraception, with lighter, less painful menstruation, and afford some protection against ascending sexually* transmitted diseases due to the effect on the cervical* mucus.

progestogens: synthetic progesterone* preparations widely used in the treatment of menstrual disorders and as one of the components of combined oral contraceptive* pills and hormone* replacement therapy preparations.

progression: the forward mobility of spermatozoa* in a semen* sample. Traditionally progression is graded on a scale from 0 (very poor) to 4 (excellent). The WHO* has recently introduced the following classification: a = rapid linear motility, b = slow, c = non-progressive, d = immotile. The fertility of a semen sample and performance during IVF* are directly related to sperm progression.

Profasi: proprietary brand of human* chorionic gonadotrophin. (See human chorionic gonadotrophin, hCG.)

prolactin: a hormone secreted from the anterior lobe of the pituitary* gland. Raised prolactin concentrations occur in pregnancy and are needed for the establishment of lactation*.

Hyperprolactinaemia* may be caused by a pituitary* adenoma*; it can also be caused by certain drugs used for the treatment of anxiety, depression and hypertension*, and can occur in hypothyroidism*.

Hyperprolactinaemia leads to the suppression of GnRH* pulsatility, causing amenorrhoea*, anovulation* and galactorrhoea* in women. In men, impotence* may be seen, but it is only a rare cause of infertility. (See hyperprolactinaemia.)

prolactinoma: a hormone* producing tumour of the pituitary* gland. (See pituitary adenoma, hyperprolactinaemia.)

pronucleate stage tubal transfer (PROST): the transfer of pronucleate*

embryos, created by *in vitro* fertilization (IVF*), to the Fallopian* tubes. This procedure is now only rarely performed.

pronucleus (Fig. 21): nucleus* present in the activated* oocyte* before syngamy*. The mature sperm* and oocyte* are haploid*. Once fertilized, the oocyte normally contains two haploid pronuclei, one derived from the fertilizing sperm and the other from the oocyte.

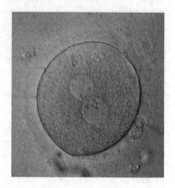

Fig. **21**. Pronucleus. Fertilized human oocyte containing two pronuclei.

Pronuclei are usually visible in human oocytes approximately 18 hours after insemination and the presence of two is regarded as evidence of successful fertilization*; numbers other than two are considered abnormal. During the later stages of fertilization, the pronuclei move together towards the centre of the oocyte, fuse, and their nucleoli* collect at the junction between the pronuclei. As the embryo enters syngamy*, the pronuclear membranes break down.

prostaglandins: a widely distributed group of locally active hormones*, synthesized from arachidonic acid. Prostaglandins have many roles in relation to inflammation, and blood vessel and platelet function. They have multiple effects on the reproductive system: PGE_2 and PGF_2 may be important in follicular* rupture and oocyte* release, regression of the corpus* luteum (and thus the onset of labour) and myometrial* contractility. They are present in high concentrations in the endometrium* and play an important role in the vasodilatation and vasoconstriction associated with menstruation*. Dysmenorrhoea* and menorrhagia* are thought to be associated with changes in the ratios of various vasoactive prostaglandins.

Intravaginal prostaglandins are used for cervical* ripening prior to termination of pregnancy and for induction of labour; systemic prostaglandins (with or without mifepristone*) are used for the medical termination of pregnancy.

In men, prostaglandins (usually PGE) are successfully used in the treatment of erectile impotence*. Self-injected direct into the corpora* cavernosa of the penis*, their action is shorter than that of papaverine*, with less likelihood of scarring.

prostaglandin synthetase inhibitors (antiprostaglandins): a large group of non-steroidal anti-inflammatory drugs (NSAID), including aspirin, indomethacin, ibuprofen and mefenamic acid. They have a wide range of clinical applications; in reproductive medicine, they may be used for the treatment of dysmenorrhoea* and menorrhagia*. Low dose aspirin has been suggested to improve the outcome of pregnancies in women with recurrent* miscarriages, pre-eclampsia* and fetal growth retardation. Indomethacin may also be used to decrease hydramnios* and to arrest uterine contractions in premature labour.

prostate (Fig. 15): a solid organ, the size of a chestnut, situated at the base of the bladder in the male, surrounding the first part of the urethra*. The prostatic secretion, which is slightly acid, normally contributes one third of the volume of the seminal* fluid.

The condition of the prostate gland can be assessed by the estimation of prostate specific antigen (PSA) concentration in serum (see prostate-specific antigen). Prostatitis, an inflammation of the gland, which may be acute, chronic or subclinical, can be a cause of male subfertility. It is commonly initiated by Chlamydia* infection and aggravated by alcohol consumption. In most elderly men, the prostate undergoes benign enlargement which may restrict the passage of urine and may ultimately require surgical treatment. Carcinoma of the prostate is one of the commonest cancers in men.

prostate-specific antigen test (PSA): a blood test performed to detect diseases of the prostate* gland. The PSA concentration in serum is raised in prostatitis, benign prostatic hypertrophy and prostatic cancer, and can be used as an annual screening test for prostate cancer in men over 50 years.

protein: a class of biochemical substances consisting of amino* acids joined together by peptide bonds to form chains. There are 20 different naturally occurring amino acids, so the number of different proteins possible is virtually infinite. Examples of proteins include enzymes*, antibodies*, haemoglobin and various structural proteins (e.g. those that make up muscle, connective tissue and hair) and certain hormones (e.g. insulin).

Proteins are synthesized in the cytoplasm* of cells* and the order of their amino acids is the result of chemical instructions carried by messenger RNA* which is made in the nucleus*. In turn, the message carried by a particular messenger RNA is determined by the order of bases found in the corresponding gene*. Generally speaking, each functioning gene codes for a single protein or part of a protein. Mutations* in genes can result in malfunctioning proteins.

pseudocyesis (phantom pregnancy, also known as hypothalamic* pregnancy): a psycho-somatic condition which may be associated with an intense desire for pregnancy, or (especially in menopausal* women) fear of pregnancy. The patient will probably have secondary amenorrhoea* (though there may be small bleeds, thought of as a threatened miscarriage*), increase in weight and abdominal distension; there may be breast changes and she is usually convinced that she can feel fetal movements. However, the pregnancy* test is negative, fetal parts are not palpable and ultrasound* scanning shows no uterine enlargement.

pseudohermaphroditism: see hermaphroditism.

psychogenic impotence: male sexual dysfunction due to a non-organic cause, for example stress or anxiety. Affected men can usually produce semen* for assisted* reproductive procedures, and usually respond to treatment with paperverine* or prostaglandin* injections. Before resorting to artificial* insemination procedures, care should be taken that there is no marital dysharmony or imminent breakdown which might affect a future child. (See impotence.)

puberty: the time in adolescence* when the sexual organs mature and secondary sexual* characteristics appear. In both sexes there is a period of rapid growth. In girls, breast enlargement and the appearance of pubic hair ususally precede the onset of menstruation*; axillary hair growth may occur later. In boys, there is deepening of the voice, growth of facial hair and development of the typical adult male hair distribution. Nocturnal ejaculation* may begin.

The onset of puberty depends on a rise of serum gonadotrophin* concentrations, stimulating the production of oestrogens* and androgens*. The rise is caused both by increased output of hypothalamic* GnRH* and by increased sensitivity of the pituitary* gland to GnRH. The age at which puberty commences has been decreasing in the last decades in some societies. This is associated with better nutrition, especially higher protein intake, and with better general health. There appears to be a critical body weight which triggers the onset of menstruation in girls. The same factor may be involved in the amenorrhoea* of women with anorexia* and highly weight conscious athletes and dancers. There is also some evidence that exposure to light affects the pituitary–hypothalamic axis and it has been suggested that more widespread electricity has increased such exposure. (See also precocious puberty.)

pulsatile GnRH therapy: the pulsatile administration of gonadotrophin* releasing hormone (GnRH), which is normally produced in the hypothalamus* and regulates gonadotrophin* synthesis from the pituitary* gland.

In the treatment of hypogonadotrophic* hypogonadism, in both men and women, a mechanical pump is used to administer small doses of subcutaneous GnRH at regular intervals in a pulsatile manner. In women, follicular* development is monitored by ultrasound* screening of the ovaries*. HCG* is needed to simulate the LH* surge. In women with polycystic* ovaries, the use of the GnRH pump is likely to produce a single follicle and avoids the risk of ovarian hyperstimulation* (OHSS) from the use of hMG*.

pyosalpinx: distension of the distal portion of the Fallopian* tube with pus. This is usually the result of ascending genital tract infection (see pelvic inflammatory disease) and is particularly likely if the abdominal* ostium is occluded (see hydrosalpinx). It can also be caused by tuberculous infection.

R

random sampling: a statistical device whereby a number of individuals (the sample) are selected from a population in such a way that each member of the population has an equal probability of being included in the sample. The sample may then be regarded as truly representative of the population. Tables of random numbers have been published to assist the investigator to implement this procedure.

randomization: a statistical procedure whereby sampling, selection, ordering, or allocation are carried out by a purely random process such as coin tossing or the selection of random numbers from a table. As applied to experimental investigations involving treatments, the allocation of the treatments to the experimental subjects such as patients or animals needs to be completely random, in order to guarantee objectivity. Randomization is generally regarded as essential for the validity of many statistical analyses*.

Reactive oxygen species (ROS): oxygen-containing molecules (e.g. hydrogen peroxide) which are collectively known as free radicals and which are involved in some physiological processes, such as the acrosome* reaction, sperm hyperactivation*, oocyte–spermatozoon binding and fertilization*. These events involve changes in cell membranes, mediated by the action of ROS on unsaturated fatty acids.

Under certain conditions, when present in excess, ROS have adverse effects, such as depression of sperm motility and fertilizing ability, and impairment of embryo growth *in vitro*. ROS concentrations are increased in the seminal* fluid of two thirds of infertile males, where they are produced by inflammatory cells and dysfunctional spermatozoa. Vitamins C and E, normally present in seminal fluid, are antioxidants which scavenge ROS and protect spermatozoa. Smoking has been shown to reduce vitamin C in seminal plasma. Pentoxifylline*, an *in vitro* sperm stimulant, is also a scavenger of ROS.

recessive: in a normal diploid* cell, the alleles* that make up a gene* are found in pairs, one allele being maternal in origin, the other paternal. An allele is said to be recessive when it only has its effect if inherited from both parents. For example, the allele responsible for cystic* fibrosis is recessive. Someone who has only one copy of the cystic fibrosis gene is perfectly healthy but is said to be a carrier for that allele. (See dominance.)

recombination: the phenomenon which takes place during meiosis* when two chromatids* break at the same place and then exchange their genetic material before the breaks are mended. This is perfectly normal. In evolution, recombination allows genes* to be swapped between maternal and paternal chromosomes*. This increases variation and is one of the reasons why no two individuals (unless they are identical twins) are genetically the same.

recombinant DNA technology: a technique used to produce pure synthetic proteins* by introducing a desired gene* sequence into a bacterium* or other host cell. The cloned DNA* is used for large scale synthesis of substances such as FSH*, LH* and growth* hormone.

recurrent miscarriage (*syn.* habitual miscarriage, recurrent/habitual abortion): the loss of three or more consecutive pregnancies before the 24th week; approximately 1 woman in 100 is affected. As at least 15% of all pregnancies result in a miscarriage* (see also early pregnancy loss), repeated miscarriage can be purely due to chance, but the more miscarriages a woman has suffered, the more likely she is to have further ones.

Among the causes of recurrent miscarriage are parental chromosomal* abnormalities; anatomical abnormalities in the genital tract, such as incomplete fusion of the Müllerian* ducts; fibroids* and cervical* incompetence. Hypersecretion of luteinizing* hormone (LH), vaginal infections (see bacterial vaginosis) and immunological factors have more recently been suggested as causative factors. One significant immunological factor is the antiphospholipid antibody syndrome, involving a coagulation defect which compromises the placental circulation. This responds well to treatment with low dose aspirin (with or without heparin) given in pregnancy. (See also lupus anticoagulant.)

Women with repeated miscarriages require a special degree of sympathy and understanding. Investigations are best performed in a dedicated clinic where general support, as well as specific treatments, can be offered for future pregnancies. Such management has an approximately 80% chance of a successful pregnancy.

refractile body: a bright structure found in the ooplasm* of some oocytes*. One, two or occasionally more may occur in a single oocyte. Refractile bodies are composed of lipid and granular material, but their origin is unknown. Oocytes with refractile bodies may recur in individual patients and are associated with a reduced fertilization* rate by conventional IVF*. ICSI* may overcome this problem.

resistant ovary syndrome: an autoimmune* disorder which is one of the causes of premature* ovarian failure. Although follicles* are present in the ovarian* cortex, FSH* fails to stimulate either oestrogen* production or follicular development. This is thought to be due to blockage of the FSH receptors. Patients have amenorrhoea*, raised FSH and low oestrogen* concentrations and normal ovarian histology. The condition can be intermittent and rare spontaneous pregnancies have been reported. However, generally these patients require hormone* replacement therapy, and egg* donation if they wish to achieve a pregnancy.

rete testis (Fig. 25): a network of tubules within the testis*, which receive spermatozoa* from the seminiferous* tubules and give rise to the efferent ducts which carry the spermatozoa to the head of the epididymis*. Rete testis obstruction, a type of intra-testicular obstructive* azoospermia, may be due to antisperm* antibodies. It can be treated with low dose steroids* or by testicular* sperm extraction (TESE) for ICSI*.

retained products of conception (RPC): placental or other pregnancy-related tissue remaining in the uterus* after incomplete miscarriage*, termination of pregnancy or delivery. In the presence of RPC, patients continue to bleed, the external* cervical os is open, and the uterus is bulky. Secondary infection can occur and antibiotics may be required prior to surgical evacuation of the uterus. The presence of RPC can be detected by ultrasound* scanning.

retrograde ejaculation: the passage of semen* into the bladder at orgasm*. This can occur spontaneously, in diabetics and in men with multiple sclerosis, due to autonomic nerve damage. It is more often the result of transurethral resection of an enlarged prostate*, of surgical interference with autonomic nerve fibres during major pelvic operations or of certain drugs, e.g. phenothiazines. For infertility treatment, spermatozoa* can be collected from alkalinized urine for AIH*.

retrograde menstruation: the passage of menstrual fluid (blood and shed endometrial* glands) along the Fallopian* tubes into the peritoneal cavity. Whilst the utero*–tubal junction is normally closed during menstruation, it is not a perfect barrier and retrograde menstruation is a common event. It can cause dysmenorrhoea* and is one of the factors involved in the pathogenesis of endometriosis*.

retroverted uterus: the position of the uterus* where the uterine body (corpus) tilts backwards and occupies the pouch* of Douglas. The cervix* points upwards and forwards. Retroversion occurs normally in about 20% of women and, if the uterus is mobile, is of no clinical significance. In pregnancy, a retroverted uterus usually rises spontaneously into the abdomen. A fixed retroversion is usually associated with adhesions* due to pelvic infections (see pelvic inflammatory disease) or endometriosis*.

In infertility investigations, a high, forward pointing cervix (behind the back of the pubic symphysis) may be out of the 'line of fire' of the ejaculate* and this would be noted by consistently negative post-coital* tests in the presence of a normal semen* analysis. Sometimes with a retroverted uterus, the ovaries prolapse into the pouch of Douglas and this can cause pain during intercourse. The resultant deep dyspareunia* can reduce both the frequency of intercourse and the degree of penetration and treatment may be necessary.

RNA (ribonucleic acid): a class of biochemical compounds made up of chains of nucleotides, each nucleotide containing ribose (a five-carbon sugar), a phosphate group and one of a number of possible nitrogenous bases. Three forms of RNA are found: ribosomal RNA (rRNA), messenger RNA (mRNA) and transfer RNA (tRNA). Essentially, RNA carries instructions from DNA* in the nucleus* to the cytoplasm* of the cell where the instructions are used to make all the various proteins* found in the cell. (See nucleic acid.)

Robertsonian translocation: one of a number of chromosome* abnormalities in which part of a chromosome is transferred to another chromosome. The great majority of people with Down's* syndrome have 47 chromosomes, possessing an extra copy of chromosome* 21, but about 4% have the normal 46 chromosomes. Such people have a Robertsonian translocation in which the extra chromosome 21 exists not as an independent chromosome but as an addition to another one (usually one of chromosome 13, 14 or 15).

The significance of Down's syndrome resulting from a Robertsonian translocation is that any siblings of the affected individual have a great likelihood (theoretically between 1 in 3 and 1 in 4) of being affected. In practice the risk is lower, i.e. 5 to 15%; this is probably due to an increased chance of miscarriage* of affected fetuses. Every baby born with Down's syndrome is studied genetically. If a Robertsonian translocation, rather than the commoner trisomy*, is found, it is even more important that prenatal* diagnosis by amniocentesis* should be offered to the mother in any subsequent pregnancy.

rubella (German measles): a virus* infection which causes a rash, often associated with swollen lymph nodes around the head and neck. In children, this is a mild illness which usually resolves within a week.

Rubella infection during pregnancy can infect the fetus (congenital rubella) with serious consequences, particularly during the early stages of gestation. Infection in the first 16 weeks is most serious and often results in fetal loss or severe congenital abnormalities affecting mainly the heart, eye and brain. Infections after 16 weeks are less serious, though hearing problems and diabetes may develop in the child.

In order to overcome congenital rubella infection, rubella vaccine was introduced in the UK in 1970. Initially, vaccination was targeted at girls aged 12 and 13 years, but now all children should be vaccinated at 15 months and 4 years. Women are screened before becoming pregnant (e.g. in infertility clinics) or in early pregnancy, and vaccination should be provided if necessary. Vaccination cannot be done in pregnancy and if a pregnant woman contracts rubella, especially in the first 16 weeks, she is tested for rubella immunity. Pregnancy termination may be offered to those who are not immune because of the high risk of foetal abnormality.

Re-infection with rubella can occur, following both natural infection and vaccination, and can cause fetal infection in about 10% of cases.

RU 486: see mifepristone.

S

salpingectomy: surgical excision of the Fallopian* tube. The indications for this include chronic salpingitis* and tubal extra-uterine* pregnancies in which conservative management is inappropriate. Bilateral salpingectomy is a form of sterilization* which can be performed by laparotomy* or by laparoscopy*.

salpingitis: inflammation of the Fallopian* tubes: this is usually bilateral, and is part of the pelvic* inflammatory disease syndrome. Infection is usually ascending and sexually transmitted, with *Chlamydia* *trachomatis* and *Neisseria* *gonorrhoea* as the common infecting organisms; it can also be blood-borne as in tubal tuberculosis*, or result from direct spread from infections within the peritoneal* cavity, such as perforated appendicitis.

Salpingitis may be acute or chronic: the latter term includes tubes exposed to recurrent infections resulting in thickened walls, intratubal adhesions*, loss of cilia* and possibly occlusion. Loss of tubal motility interferes with the ovum* pick-up mechanism at ovulation* and with the transport of gametes*. Even if the tubes remains patent, infertility* is likely, and, if conception should occur, extra-uterine* pregnancy occurs frequently. (See pelvic inflammatory disease.)

salpingitis isthmica nodosa (SIN): the condition in which the proximal part (intramural portion and isthmus) of the Fallopian* tube becomes thickened and indurated and develops small cystic lesions outside the lumen, but in connection with it. SIN is diagnosed by X-rays (hystero-salpingography*, using a low viscosity, water soluble contrast medium) and is also known as tubal diverticulosis. Palpation of the affected portion of the tube during open surgery, or at laparoscopy, may also point to the diagnosis.

There is some dispute about the aetiology, but both chronic inflammatory changes (especially following gonococcal* infection) and endometriosis can produce SIN. Infertility* and extra-uterine* tubal pregnancy may occur. Tubal surgery is contra-indicated and infertility treatment is by IVF*.

salpingography: see hystero-salpingography.

salpingolysis: surgical procedure to free the Fallopian* tube(s) from adhesions* in order to restore fertility. The adhesions usually follow episodes of salpingitis* and occur between the tubes and uterus*, ovaries* and broad* ligaments. Salpingolysis is performed by open microsurgery* or operative laparoscopy*. Success depends on the extent and severity of the adhesions and associated tubal damage, and, in severe cases, IVF* is the treatment of choice to restore fertility.

salpingo-oophorectomy: surgical excision of the Fallopian* tube and ovary*: this may be necessary in the treatment of ovarian tumours or chronic inflammatory disease involving both tube and ovary. In ovarian or uterine cancer, bilateral salpingo-oophorectomy (BSO) is usually performed. BSO is also done routinely by most gynaecologists at the time of hysterectomy* in post-menopausal* women in order to prevent the possible development of ovarian* cancer.

salpingo-oophoritis: inflammation* involving both the Fallopian* tubes and ovaries* (see salpingitis, pelvic inflammatory disease). Salpingo-oophoritis may be acute or chronic. In acute cases, especially if treatment is delayed or incomplete, pelvic peritonitis, pyosalpinx* or tubo-ovarian* abscess may occur and cause severe illness and subsequent infertility.

salpingo-ovariolysis: surgical operation to remove adhesions* involving the Fallopian* tubes and ovaries* in order to restore fertility. Success depends on the nature of the original infecting organism and on the density and extent of the adhesions. (See salpingolysis.)

salpingoplasty: general term applied to reconstructive surgery to the fimbrial end of the Fallopian* tubes. (See fimbrioplasty, salpingostomy.)

salpingoscopy: assessment of the endosalpinx* by passing a thin, flexible endoscope* down the operating channel of a laparoscope*, through the abdominal* ostium into the tubal ampulla*. This allows inspection of the endosalpinx and detection of any intra-luminal adhesions*. Salpingoscopy helps in the selection of patients with tubal infertility for treatment by surgery or IVF*.

salpingostomy (*syn.* neosalpingostomy): surgical operation to open the occluded fimbrial end of a hydrosalpinx*. The operation can be performed by open microsurgery*, but operative laparoscopy is now more generally employed. It is one of the commonest types of tubal reconstructive surgery. In young women, provided the tubes are not grossly disfigured by chronic salpingitis and pelvic adhesions are not too dense, the results of salpingostomy are good. In carefully selected cases IVF* can thus be avoided.

salpingotomy: incision through the outer layers of the the Fallopian* tube into its lumen to shell out a tubal (extrauterine*) pregnancy. This conservative approach to an ectopic pregnancy preserves the tube and there have been successful pregnancies subsequently. The operation is not performed if the tube is grossly distorted following tubal rupture, nor if the patient's general condition is unstable: salpingectomy* is then the operation of choice. Salpingotomy is performed either through the laparoscope* or by open surgery.

screening: the testing of whole populations or specific population groups. Mass chest radiography screening for tuberculosis has been applied to whole populations; cervical cytology* screening is done for women in certain age groups for the prevention of cervical cancer. Guthrie tests are performed on new-born infants to detect phenylketonuria* and Ashkenazi Jewish populations may be screened for Tay–Sachs* disease. In antenatal clinics, women are screened for rubella* and syphilis* and fetuses for Down's* syndrome, sickle*-cell disease and beta-thalassaemia*.

In infertility clinics, women are screened for rubella*, and usually both partners for HIV* and hepatitis* B and C. As more and more tests become available to detect specific diseases and abnormalities, difficult decisions have to be taken about their use for routine screening: both the cost–benefit ratio and the emotional stress suffered by patients have to be considered. The term screening does not apply to family-based investigations for familial* diseases (see genetic counselling).

scrotum (Fig. 15): the pouch which houses the testicles* of men. Developmentally the scrotum is the fused analogue of the two female labia* majora. Satisfactory spermatogenesis* requires a lower temperature than that within the abdominal cavity. Testicular temperature control is achieved by heat dispersion through the skin of the scrotum as well as by the mechanism to raise or lower the testicles through the action of the dartos and cremasteric muscles.

semen: see seminal fluid.

semen analysis: see seminal fluid analysis.

semen preparation: see sperm preparation.

seminal fluid: the sperm-containing, creamy fluid, volume 2 to 5 ml, ejaculated* from the penis* at orgasm*. Seminal fluid is formed from the seminal* plasma, secreted mainly by the seminal* vesicles and prostate*, and contains spermatozoa*, produced in the testes*. At ejaculation seminal fluid coagulates (clots) immediately. During coitus*, the coagulum adheres to the cervix*, protecting the spermatozoa from acid vaginal secretions, and, in some animal species, against intrusion of spermatozoa from another male. Seminal fluid liquefies *in vitro* within 20 to 30 minutes, after which seminal* fluid analysis can be performed.

seminal fluid analysis (SFA): *syn.* semen analysis, sperm count, male fertility test (MFT): the scientific analysis* of seminal* fluid, carried out to investigate male fertility or the effectiveness of vasectomy*. The technique and range of normal values have been standardized by the WHO*.

The patient must abstain from coitus for 3 days before the test and produce the sample by masturbation; the container must be kept warm and reach the laboratory within one hour. By this time, the fluid will have liquefied and the volume, viscosity, sperm concentration, motility, progression* and morphology* are determined. The specimen is searched for the presence of leucocytes and immature sperm forms, and tested for antisperm* antibodies by either the MAR* or Immunobead* test.

The SFA seeks to measure the fertility potential of the man, but its accuracy is questionable due to the occurrence of occult sperm* dysfunction.

seminal plasma: the fluid part of the semen*, normally 2–5 ml, which acts as transport medium for spermatozoa*. It is a complex, slightly alkaline fluid, about two thirds derived from the seminal* vesicles, one third from the prostate* gland and with small contributions from the testes*, epididymes* and bulbo-urethral (Cowper's) glands.

Chemical analysis of specific substances in the seminal plasma, produced by its individual contributing glands, can be utilized as biochemical markers of gland function; for example fructose* is produced by the seminal* vesicles, acid phophatase by the prostate* and alpha-glucosidase by the epididymides*.

seminal vesicles (Fig. 15): a pair of multilobular glands, situated at the base of the bladder, above and behind the prostate* gland. The seminal vesicles have ducts which join the ampulla of the vas* to form the ejaculatory* ducts. They contribute two thirds of the volume of the seminal* plasma and secrete fructose*, prostaglandins* and fibrin. Seminal vesicle fluid is alkaline.

seminiferous tubules (Fig. 25): the highly tortuous, fine tubules of the testis* which manufacture spermatozoa*. Each testis contains about 500 seminiferous tubules, gathered into lobules. The tubules are arranged as loops within the lobules and straighten before converging on the mediastinum of the testis where they amalgamate to form the rete* testis. Seminiferous tubules are lined by Sertoli* cells which nurture and support spermatogenesis* under endocrine* control.

sensitivity: one of a pair of terms (see also specificity) used in medical investigations to quantify the performance of a test procedure. Sensitivity defines the probability that a test procedure will correctly identify a condition which is present. It is therefore very similar to the 'power' of a statistical test, which is the more familiar term in the standard statistical literature. The difference of the sensitivity value from unity, which represents the failure to detect a condition which is present, is often referred to as 'false negative'.

Sertoli cells: the lining cells of the seminiferous* tubules, sensitive to FSH*, which control and nurture spermatogenesis*.

Sertoli-cell-only syndrome (del Castillo syndrome): a form of primary testicular* failure with azoospermia*. The seminiferous* tubules are small and contain only Sertoli* cells with no sperm-producing germ cells. The testes* are usually small and atrophic and the serum FSH* concentration is grossly elevated. Apart from the infertility, affected men appear as normal males.

The aetiology of this syndrome is not known, but genetic abnormalities, late testicular descent and viral or toxic damage to the testes have been invoked. In about 50% of men with Sertoli-cell-only syndrome, multiple small testicular biopsies* reveal minute isolated nests of normal spermatogenesis* and from these testicular spermatozoa may be successfully extracted for ICSI*.

sex chromatin: the DNA* and proteins* that make up the X* and Y* chromosomes*. (See Barr body.)

sex chromosomes: the X and Y chromosomes* which determine the sex of an individual. (See also sex determination, sex-linked abnormalities, X and Y chromosomes.)

sex determination: in humans, a person's sex is determined by the balance of their sex* chromosomes. A normal female has two X* chromosomes (i.e. her chromosome complement is XX plus 44 non-sex chromosomes), a normal male has an X and a Y* chromosome (i.e. his chromosome complement is XY plus 44 non-sex chromosomes). It is the presence of a gene on the Y chromosome which confers masculinity. Thus individuals who have only one X chromosome and no Y chromosome (XO, Turner's* syndrome) are female (albeit infertile), whilst those with an XXY complement (Klinefelter's* syndrome) are male (and also infertile).

sex-linked abnormalities: inherited disorders, such as red–green colour blindness, Duchenne's* muscular dystrophy and haemophilia*, in which the gene* concerned is located on the X* chromosome. Most sex-linked disorders are recessive*. This means that females, who have two X chromosomes, need two copies of the affected allele* to show the disorder. However, as males, unlike females, have only a single X chromosome, they show the disorder if they carry just one copy of the affected allele. (The presence of the Y chromosome can be ignored as it carries almost no genes.) This means that sex-linked abnormalities are much more often seen in males than females.
   Females can be carriers of the allele, which means that they possess one normal copy and one faulty copy of the gene in question, but show no clinical signs of the abnormality themselves. If a woman who is a carrier has a partner who is unaffected by the disorder, there is a 50% chance that any sons they have will be affected with the disorder. None of their daughters will be affected but, on average, half of them will be carriers.

sexual characteristics: the primary sexual characteristics are the presence of the penis* or vulva* and are present from birth. Newborn male and female infants are distinguished by the appearance of their external genitalia. The secondary sexual characteristics appear at puberty* and include a generalized bodily growth spurt and maturation of the genital tract in both sexes. In girls, breast development, pubic and axillary

hair growth and menstruation commence. In boys there are facial, pubic and axillary hair growth, voice changes and, often, noctural ejaculation*.

sexually transmitted disease (STD): diseases in which sexual contact is the usual mode of transmission. They include the statutory venereal diseases—syphilis*, gonorrhoea* and chancroid—as well as chlamydial* infection, non-specific urethritis, viral infections such as hepatitis B*, herpes*, human* papilloma virus and human* immunodeficiency virus, and parasitic infections such as scabies and pubic lice. Specific clinics for the diagnosis and treatment of STDs, where confidentiality* is paramount, exist throughout the UK. Contact* tracing is a very important part of the work carried out in these clinics.

Sheehan's syndrome: see postpartum pituitary necrosis.

Shirodkar operation: operation performed to narrow the calibre of the cervical* canal in cases of cervical* incompetence. Incompetence can result from difficult delivery, overdilatation* of the cervix and other operations on the cervix or be associated with congenital abnormalities of the uterus. Repeated second trimester* miscarriages or premature labours, with painless expulsion of a normal fetus, may result from cervical incompetence. The operation is usually performed vaginally towards the end of the first trimester of a normal pregnancy and consists of the insertion of a submucosal suture around the cervix. The suture is removed a short time before term and spontaneous onset of labour usually follows.

sickle-cell disease: the family of recessively* inherited haemoglobin disorders having in common the inheritance of the sickle gene* from one, or both, parents. While the homozygous* SS state is the most common, the second abnormal β globin gene can also be another variant, e.g. haemoglobin C, giving rise to haemoglobin SC disease or a β thalassaemia* gene, giving rise to haemoglobin S β thalassaemia. The sickle mutation is found in sub-Saharan Africans, Arabs, Indians and people from the Mediterranean. Ante-natal screening* by chorionic* villus sampling may be offered to women at risk of producing an affected infant.

sickle test: a laboratory screening* blood test for the presence of sickle haemoglobin. A positive sickle test does not distinguish between healthy sickle-cell trait carriers and those with sickle*-cell disease. Haemoglobin electrophoresis should always be performed in order to determine the full haemoglobin phenotype*.

single cell biopsy: see pre-implantation diagnosis.

single gene defect: see gene disorder.

smoking: smoking decreases the amount of oxygen available to the body and adversely affects respiratory function, the immune system and blood coagulability. In women, tobacco smoking has increased dramatically in recent decades. Nicotine is an anti*-oestrogen and a potential carcinogen, and there is a positive relationship between smoking and cancer of the cervix*. In pregnancy, women who smoke have an increased incidence of miscarriage*, premature labour, placental abruption and growth retarded babies. Women who smoke are also at higher risk of thrombosis* when taking oral contraceptives and when having surgery. Advice on stopping smoking is an important part of preconceptual counselling and antenatal care.

In men, tobacco smoking can lead to the reduction of the antioxidant activity of the seminal* fluid (due to depletion of Vitamin C) and may interfere with the acrosome* reaction. However, male fertility is probably affected more by high alcohol consumption than by smoking.

somatic cell: any cell in the body except for the gametes*. Somatic cells have a diploid* number of chromosomes*, i.e. 46 in humans. Mutations* can occur during somatic cell division (mitosis*), but these are not passed on to any offspring.

specificity: one of a pair of terms (see also sensitivity) used in medical investigations to quantify the performance of a test procedure. Specificity defines the probability that a test procedure will correctly fail to detect a condition when it is absent. The difference of the specificity value from unity, which represents the erroneous detection of a condition when it is absent, is called 'false positive'. This statistic is variously described as error of the first kind, Alpha type error, P value, or the size of a test, in statistical texts. The size of a test may be adjusted in order to increase specificity, but only by decreasing sensitivity, or vice versa.

speculum: an instrument, metal or plastic, used in gynaecological practice, to expose the cervix* for inspection, taking of cervical* smears, operations on the cervix, sounding the uterine cavity, insertion of IUCDs* and artificial* insemination. Specula are 'bivalve' or have a single lower blade only with a special retraction handle (Sim's) or a weighted appendage (Auvard's).

sperm: see spermatozoon.

sperm antibodies: see antisperm antibodies.

sperm–cervical mucus contact test (SCMC): see sperm–mucus interaction.

sperm count (sperm concentration): the number of spermatozoa present in 1 ml of seminal fluid*. A count is performed by microscope in the laboratory using a Makler* chamber, Neubauer* haemocytometer or a computerized system.

The WHO* definition of a 'normal' sperm count is 20 million or more per ml; patients with persistently lower counts are considered subfertile. The total sperm count is the total number of spermatozoa in a single ejaculate. The total motile sperm count is calculated by multiplying the total sperm count by the sperm motility, and a value of 20 million motile spermatozoa per ejaculate is considered normal.

Sperm dysfunction: the condition when spermatozoa* are unable to fertilize oocytes*. Sperm dysfunction is the largest cause of male infertility, but in most cases the cause is unknown. A man with a normal seminal* fluid analysis with no evidence of anti-sperm* antibodies may still be infertile due to sperm dysfunction. The condition is diagnosed by failure of fertilization during IVF* or by specialized sperm* function tests. In clinical practice, if there has been failed fertilization, ICSI* is usually performed, making unnecessary the performance of further sperm function tests.

sperm function tests: methods for the laboratory diagnosis of defective sperm function, also known as diagnostic andrology studies, which seek to assess the fertilizing potential of spermatozoa* in order to predict the outcome of fertility treatment, particularly IVF*. Such tests include analysis of sperm activity (sperm survival *in vitro*, CASA*, hyperactivation*), strict* sperm morphology* criteria (WHO* or Kruger), cervical mucus penetration tests (see PCT*, SCMC* test, Kremer* penetration test), sperm–oocyte interaction (hemi-zona assay), the acrosome* reaction (ARIC*), zona-free hamster* oocyte penetration test and biochemical tests for reactive* oxygen species (ROS) and creatinine phosphokinase (CPK).

The variety of tests developed reflects the diversity of biological functions which have been developed by the highly differentiated sperm cell in order to enable it to locate, become selected and then fertilize a single oocyte* within the female reproductive tract.

sperm reservoir: an artificially established source of spermatozoa* which can be tapped intermittently in assisted* reproductive technology, used in obstructive* azoospermia and aspermia* (ejaculatory failure, e.g. spinal injury). Attempts to establish sperm reservoirs by surgically creating artificial* spermatoceles or implanting plastic devices for tapping through the scrotum* have generally been abandoned in favour of instant surgical* sperm retrieval for ICSI*.

spermatic cord: the bundle of vessels, nerves and muscle which connects each testicle* to the body, through the inguinal canal in the groin, and thereby suspends the testis* within the scrotum*. The spermatic cord contains the vas* deferens, three arteries*, the pampiniform plexus of veins*, lymphatic vessels, sympathetic nerves, the blind-ending upper extension of the tunica* vaginalis, connective tissue and also some fibres of the cremaster muscle which draw the testicle into the inguinal canal during heavy exercise or threat of injury.

The close proximity of the testicular artery and the pampiniform plexus creates a biological countercurrent mechanism which is involved in heat and metabolic exchanges, thereby preserving the correct low temperature and physiological environment within the testis for optimum sperm production. (See spermatogenesis.)

spermatid (Fig. 22): immature sperm cell with half the normal number of chromosomes* (haploid*). Spermatids are the final stage of cell division during spermatogenesis*. Initially rounded cells, they elongate and by a process of metamorphosis (spermiogenesis*) develop into spermatozoa* without further division.

Maturation arrest at the spermatid stage is one cause of arrested spermatogenesis* and azoospermia*. Some spermatids may reach the semen*. Spermatids obtained from testis* or semen have been used for ICSI*, but this treatment is currently not permitted by the HFEA* in the UK.

spermatocele: an asymptomatic retention cyst* of the epididymis*, efferent duct or rete* testis, which contains spermatozoa*. Spermatoceles occur in about 1% of men; they are usually small and unobtrusive; if found in men with irreversible obstructive* azoopermia, simple needle aspiration, without local anaesthesia, can provide sufficient spermatozoa for ICSI*.(See also artificial spermatocele, sperm reservoir.)

spermatogenesis (Fig. 22): the complex process of multiple cell divisions resulting in sperm* formation within the seminiferous* tubules of the testis*. Spermatogenesis, under the influence of the pituitary* gonadotrophic* hormones (FSH* and LH*), commences at puberty* and continues throughout life. Spermatogonia*, the stem* cells, divide to give rise to daughter

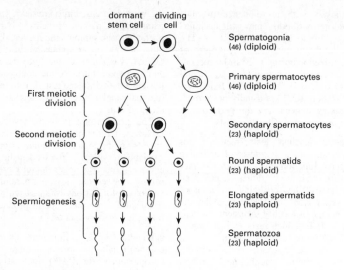

dormant   dividing
stem cell   cell

Spermatogonia
(46) (diploid)

First meiotic
division

Primary spermatocytes
(46) (diploid)

Second meiotic
division

Secondary spermatocytes
(23) (haploid)

Round spermatids
(23) (haploid)

Spermiogenesis

Elongated spermatids
(23) (haploid)

Spermatozoa
(23) (haploid)

Fig. **22**. The Stages of Spermatogenesis.

cells, which undergo meiosis*, passing though primary and secondary spermatocyte stages, to give rise to haploid* spermatids* which do not divide further, but develop, by a process of metamorphosis, into fully-formed spermatozoa*. The entire process of spermatogenesis is nurtured by the Sertoli* cells and takes about 70 days in man. Normally a man produces at least 20 million spermatozoa per day, and, on average, most men would ejaculate about a billion spermatozoa per month. (See also spermiogenesis.)

Spermatogenesis, and therefore male fertility, may be arrested by occupational or other environmental hazards, e.g. increased heat in the work place (welders, furnace worker, drivers due to prolonged sitting), exposure to toxic chemicals (some insecticides, lead, mercury, cadmium), irradiation (nuclear workers, X-ray personnel), testicular conditions (orchitis*, undescended* testes, torsion, varicocele*), alcohol*, some drugs (see drug effects on fertility) and radiotherapy (e.g. for testicular cancer, lymphoma).

spermatogonia (Fig. 22): the diploid* stem* cells within the seminiferous* tubules of the testis*, which are the precursors of spermatozoa*. Situated at the base of the seminiferous tubules, surrounded by Sertoli* cells, they

undergo division into spermatocytes, which undergo meiosis* to produce spermatids* and ultimately the spermatozoa.

spermatozoon (*pl.* spermatozoa; Fig. 23): the male gamete*, produced in the testis* and transported through the genital tract into the semen*. Spermatozoa are highly specialized cells, adapted to carry the genetic male contribution of DNA* through the female reproductive tract and to locate and fertilize the oocyte*. Spermatozoa have a head (containing the acrosome* and the haploid* number of chromosomes*), a mid-piece (containing mitochondria* which power the tail), and a tail or flagellum which has a central core mechanism, the axoneme, and confers motility.

spermiogenesis: the process of metamorphosis, occurring during the final stages of spermatogenesis*, whereby round spermatids* elongate and become transformed into recognisable spermatozoa* with heads and tails, without further cell division.

sperm–mucus interaction: investigation of this process is an important part of infertility investigations. The postcoital* test (PCT) is the most basic study of the sperm–mucus relationship. It provides information about the

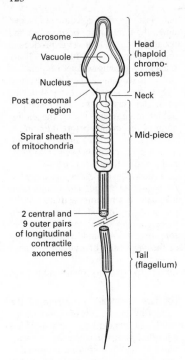

Acrosome

Vacuole

Nucleus

Post acrosomal region

Spiral sheath of mitochondria

2 central and 9 outer pairs of longitudinal contractile axonemes

Head (haploid chromosomes)

Neck

Mid-piece

Tail (flagellum)

Fig. 23. Spermatozoon: detailed structure.

quality and receptiveness of the cervical* mucus and the density, motility, morphology and behaviour of the spermatozoa*. Persistently negative PCTs, (i.e. few or no spermatozoa, or absence of motility) indicate an abnormality of the mucus or of the semen, or difficulty with coitus. In doubtful cases, *in vitro* sperm–mucus penetration tests may be used, in which a specimen of cervical mucus is exposed on a microscope slide or in a small test tube to a sample of semen. Bovine mucus or synthetic mucus substitute can be used instead of human mucus to assess the penetrating capacity of the spermatozoa. (See sperm function tests, Kremer test.)

sperm penetration assay (SPA): the zona*-free hamster* oocyte penetration assay, performed to test the fertilizing ability of spermatozoa*. Human spermatozoa are incubated with hamster oocytes* from which the zona* pellucida has been removed. Normal functioning spermatozoa will penetrate the oolemma*. A score, derived from the number of penetrations, is related

to the fertility of the semen sample under test.

Prior to the use of ICSI*, an inadequate score in the SPA was one of the most important methods of diagnosing sperm* dysfunction. The SPA is now not widely used in clinical practice, but is still a useful research procedure. (See also sperm function tests, sperm–mucus interaction, Kremer test.)

sperm preparation: method of producing the final sample of spermatozoa*, by extraction and purification from semen* by various laboratory techniques, to be used as the insemination sample for assisted* reproductive procedures. The methods used include layering, centrifugation and washing, swim-up, sedimentation, glass wool or glass bead columns, density* gradients or albumin* gradients.

sperm separation: method of selecting sperm populations which carry particular genetic characteristics. A variety of techniques have been used in attempts to separate spermatozoa carrying the X* and Y* chromosomes, so that insemination can be performed with a sperm population to produce male or female offspring.

In the UK, it is recommended by the HFEA* that sperm sexing be carried out only to avoid sex-linked* genetic disorders. However the practice of sex selection for other reasons is not covered by present legislation and is therefore not illegal. In some animals (cattle, sheep), sex selection can be carried out using fluorescent probes bound to spermatozoa, followed by selection according to the colour of the sperm head using a fluorescence-activated cell sorter. This method is fairly reliable, but the potential toxicity of the probes so far renders it inappropriate for humans. Other, non-toxic, methods have been tried in humans, but these are less effective, possibly providing only a slight enrichment of X or Y populations, and it is often disputed whether they work at all. Such methods include separation of spermatozoa on columns of albumin.

spina bifida: a developmental abnormality of the bones of the spinal column with a fusion defect of the vertebral arches. This can allow protrusion of the spinal cord and its membranes (meninges). The likelihood of this and the resulting symptoms depend on the extent of the fusion defect. In the mildest cases (spina bifida occulta) there is no skin defect, no protrusion of the cord or membranes, and no clinical abnormality. There may be just a dimple in the skin over the defect, or the condition is picked up incidentally on an X-ray. At the other extreme, there may be a large skin defect with extensive herniation through it of the cord and its covering membranes. Infection, leading to meningitis and encephalitis, is an immediate risk and there may be paralysis of the lower limbs and incontinence of urine and faeces. There may be an associated hydrocephalus.

In severe cases, there is a raised alpha-feto* protein concentration in the maternal serum and the fluid obtained by amniocentesis*. Ultrasound* scans show the defect. Antenatal diagnosis enables parents to consider the question of pregnancy termination in severe cases.

There are marked variations in the incidence of spina bifida in different parts of the world (it is rare in the Far East and common in Western Europe) and at different times of the year. The aetiology is almost certainly multifactorial with a genetic and an environmental component. Women who have had one child with spina bifida have an increased risk of another. This risk is reduced by the administration of small doses of folic* acid to the mother, and such medication has also been shown to be effective in reducing the over-all incidence. To be effective, medication has to be taken at a very early stage of pregnancy (4 to 6 weeks) before the neural arches are completely formed: most women do not yet know they are pregnant at this stage, and it is therefore advisable that folic acid should be taken when a woman plans to start a pregnancy. (See also neural tube defect, anencephaly.)

spinal injury: in the context of reproductive medicine, spinal injury in men may be a cause of ejaculation* failure and impotence*. (See also paraplegia and electro-ejaculation.)

spinnbarkeit (SBK): the property of the cervical* mucus to vary the viscosity and elasticity of its constituent mucins, under the influence of oestrogens* and progesterone*. Oestrogens produce a more profuse, clear, fluid and elastic mucus which allows sperm* penetration. These changes can be observed by pulling a sample of cervical mucus from the cervix with small spongeholder forceps and noting the elongation of the strands before they break. SBK can also be measured by placing a sample of mucus between two glass slides and pulling them apart.

A good quality mucus is essential for sperm penetration and results from adequate oestrogenic activity in the pre-ovulatory period. In some women these changes occur several days before ovulation*, and in others only at the very time of ovulation. These differences may partially account for the relative fertility of different individuals.

standard deviation: a measure of the variability among a set of observations. Unlike the standard error*, with which it is often confused, increasing the sample size does not effect a progressive reduction in the standard deviation, but simply provides a more reliable estimate of its value.

standard error: a measure of the reliability of a statistical estimate, perhaps derived from a random sample of observations drawn from a population. Increasing the sample size leads to a progressive reduction in the standard error. The term is often confused with standard* deviation. In order to calculate the confidence* limits from the standard error, distributional assumptions need to be made.

statistical analysis: any numerical evaluation and presentation of data. However, in biological research work the term is generally used in a narrower sense, referring to the procedure of identifying and quantifying systematic factors which influence the experimental material, in the presence of random variation.

Stein–Leventhal syndrome: the association of infertility*, obesity*, oligomenorrhoea* or amenorrhoea* and hirsutism*, with the presence of polycystic* ovaries. Since the original description of the S–L syndrome in 1935, it has been realized that the symptomatology merely represents one extreme of the wide spectrum of clinical conditions associated with polycystic ovarian syndrome. (See polycystic ovarian syndrome.)

stem cell: a self-renewing, undifferentiated cell* which can produce, by division, one or more differentiated daughter cells. When the stem cell divides, one of the two daughter cells normally remains a stem cell (maintaining the stem cell line), whilst the other daughter cell may give rise to one or more other types of cell. Many stem cells are present in embryos, and some persist into adult life to maintain cell production in certain organs; for example, the haemopoietic (blood-forming) stem cells in the bone marrow continually replace blood cells and platelets, some of which have only a short life span (120 days for red blood cells). Stem cells may be totipotential, i.e. capable of forming any type of cell, or pluripotential, i.e. capable of forming a limited number of cell types.

sterilization: the process of making an individual incapable of producing offspring. Castration*, the removal of the ovaries* or testes*, has such an effect but is not performed for routine sterilization because it would also entail the loss of the hormone-producing function of the gonads*. Sterilization in both sexes is therefore effected by interrupting the ducts which transport the gametes*, i.e. the Fallopian* tubes and vas* deferens.

Female sterilization can be performed by a wide variety of operative procedures (open or laparoscopic) on the Fallopian* tubes, ranging from total or partial excision and diathermy coagulation to the application of 'clips'. It may be performed at the time of another operation such as Caesarean section. Male sterilization is performed by dividing the vas deferens on both sides (vasectomy*), usually carried out under local anaesthesia. Possible reversal of sterilization depends in both sexes on how much viable tube or vas is left, involves major surgery and has variable success rates.

Sterilization is also the term used to describe the process of rendering something free from contamination.

sterility: inability to have children due to absence or loss of function of the gonads* or other genital organs. Causes include surgical sterilization*, hysterectomy*, removal of both gonads for malignancies, irradiation and chemotherapy. Some cases of female sterility may be treated by egg* donation. (See infertility.)

steroids: a large group of hormones*, derived from cholesterol and produced in various endocrine* glands. The sex steroids are the androgens*, oestrogens* and progesterone*. Corticosteroids are produced in the adrenal* glands. The secretion of steroids is stimulated by peptide hormones from the pituitary* gland, or, in pregnancy, by trophoblastic* hormones.

Circulating steroids are mainly bound to albumin or specific binding hormones; only the free hormones are biologically active, stimulating nuclear receptors to produce proteins* (e.g. enzymes*). Steroids, such as the corticosteroid dexamethasone, are administered to women about to give birth prematurely, in order to stimulate surfactant production and maturation of the lungs of immature babies. Steroids have also been used in the treatment of antisperm* antibodies.

stilboestrol: see diethyl stilboestrol.

stillbirth: a baby delivered after the 24th week of pregnancy which shows no sign of life. The stillbirth rate is the number of stillbirths per 1000 total births. In 1995 the combined stillbirth and first week neonatal (i.e. the perinatal) mortality* rate was approximately 8/1000 in the UK.

Important causes of stillbirth include congenital abnormalities, intra-uterine growth retardation, often associated with pre-eclampsia* or diabetes*, antepartum haemorrhage, anoxia or trauma during delivery and complications associated with the umbilical* cord. In cases of stillbirth, death certificates are issued and the mother is eligible for maternity leave. (See also mortality rates.)

stimulation (ovarian): see ovarian stimulation.

Strassman operation: an abdominal operation performed to correct uterine abnormalities, resulting from Müllerian* duct fusion failures. The purpose is to fashion a single uterine cavity from a septate or bicornuate* uterus. This operation is now no longer performed as the hysteroscopic* approach is easier and quicker, with a shorter convalescence and less likelihood of adhesion* formation. (See also Müllerian duct.)

strict criteria: a highly specialized method of defining sperm morphology* (structure) described by Kruger (Kruger criteria), whereby any sperm cell which shows any degree of variation from normal is classified as abnormal. A normal semen sample will thus contain 4% or more normal forms according to the strict criteria. This has been related to sperm fertilizing ability during IVF*. Thus if there are less than 4% normal forms, failure of fertilization* or poor fertilization can be predicted and ICSI* is indicated. The WHO* method of sperm morphology assessment has a cut-off level of 30% normal forms, since the criteria for normality are less rigid.

submucous fibroid: see fibroid.

subserous fibroid: see fibroid.

subzonal sperm insemination (SUZI): (Fig. 1.3): micro-manipulation* technique for the insertion of one or more spermatozoa* into the perivitelline* space of an oocyte*. This is performed to promote fertilization *in vitro* in cases of severe male factor infertility. Whilst a moderately successful technique in its day, it has largely been superseded by the more successful intra-cytoplasmic* sperm injection (ICSI). (See also assisted fertilization.)

superovulation: see ovarian stimulation.

surgical sperm retrieval (Fig. 24): collective term for techniques to obtain spermatozoa in obstructive* azoospermia and ejaculatory* failure (aspermia*). (See MESA, spermatocele, sperm reservoir, PESA, TESA, TESE, rete testis, vas aspiration.)

surrogacy: a procedure where a woman (the surrogate or host) carries a child for another couple (the

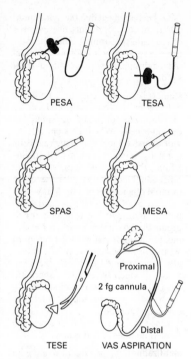

Fig. 24. Surgical Sperm Retrieval. Techniques used to obtain sperm for ICSI in azoospermia: PESA – percutaneous epididmal sperm aspiration; TESA – testicular sperm aspiration; SPAS – spermatocele aspiration; MESA – microsurgical epididmal sperm aspiration; TESE – testicular sperm extraction (from a biopsy); Vas deference aspiration.

commissioning couple). As a result of developments in reproductive technology, surrogacy has become a comparatively simple procedure which, however, raises many ethical, emotional and legal problems. In all cases, expert counselling* of all parties should be undertaken and cases may be referred to a local ethics* committee for review.

The Human* Fertilisation and Embryology Act permits surrogacy, but points out that no surrogacy arrangement is binding under British law; a change in parentage (Section 30) can take place provided that the commissioning couple are married, over 18, genetically related to the child, the host (and her husband if married) have given their consent, the applicants are domiciled in the UK, and that no money (other than expenses approved by the court) has been paid.

Surrogacy can be undertaken by artificial* insemination or by IVF* and ET*. In artificial insemination cases, the spermatozoa of the commissioning father are used so that the surrogate host carries a child which is genetically half hers and half that of the commissioning couple. This should be undertaken under proper medical supervision, but in many cases DIY (do it yourself) insemination or intercourse is used. In IVF–ET surrogacy, the embryo is entirely from the commissioning couple and is transferred to the uterus of the host: the child then has no genetic relationship to the host or her husband/partner.

The main indications for surrogacy are previous hysterectomy, repeated IVF failures, recurrent* miscarriages, pregnancy contra-indications and congenital absence of the uterus. Surrogate hosts may be friends or relatives of the commissioning couple, or may have been introduced through counsellors or support groups.

syncytiotrophoblast: the outer layer of cells lining the chorionic* villi. These cells are not only concerned with the exchange of metabolites, gases and nutrients between the fetal and maternal circulation, but also have a metabolic function of their own, i.e. the synthesis of chorionic* gonadotrophin. (See also cytotrophoblast, chorion.)

syndrome: a collection of various symptoms and clinical or laboratory signs which form a particular condition; for example, the symptoms of obesity*, amenorrhoea*, infertility* and hirsutism*, together with the ultrasound* finding of multiple peripheral follicles* and a thickened central stroma in the ovaries*, and the laboratory finding of a raised LH* concentration, make up the clinical condition known as Stein*–Leventhal syndrome. In the clinical presentation of a syndrome, any one feature may often be present in only some of the patients.

syngamy: the process in which maternal and paternal chromosomes* in the fertilized oocyte* pair in preparation to undergo the first cleavage* division. Syngamy occurs after the pronuclear membranes have broken down and the pronuclei* have disappeared.

syphilis: a serious, potentially fatal, but curable sexually* transmitted disease, caused by the spirochaete *Treponema pallidum*. Initially a painless ulcer (primary chancre) may appear on the vulva* or penis*. Secondary syphilis is the systemic manifestation of further spread with a flu-like illness, rash, enlarged lymph glands and mucosal ulcers. Tertiary syphilis with its cardiovascular and neurological sequelae is now rarely seen. Screening* for syphilis is routinely carried out during pregnancy and treatment with penicillin before the 20th week will protect the fetus from the risks of miscarriage*, stillbirth* or congenital syphilis.

T

Tamoxifen: anti-oestrogen* drug, widely used in the long term management of patients with carcinoma of the breast. Tamoxifen does have some oestrogenic properties and so stimulates the endometrium* which may lead to the growth of endometrial polyps* and post-menopausal bleeding. It gives some protection against osteoporosis* and heart disease in women after the menopause*. It is also occasionally used for the treatment of anovulatory* infertility, but clomiphene* citrate, another anti-oestrogen, is more widely used for this. Tamoxifen has, in the past, been widely prescribed for the treatment of male infertility, but this has not been proved to be beneficial. (See also oestrogens.)

TAT test: test used to detect antisperm* antibodies in the blood (serum). A titre of 1 in 32, or more, is positive and confirms the presence of sperm antibodies when there is a positive MAR* or immunobead* test for antibodies on the sperm surface.

Tay–Sachs disease: an autosomal* recessive* disease which causes mental retardation, blindness, fits and paralysis in infants, leading to death in early childhood. This metabolic abnormality, due to an inability to produce the enzyme hexosaminidase A, is common in Ashkenazi Jews. Carriers of the abnormal gene can be identified by screening* for pre-marital genetic* counselling. Antenatal diagnosis can be performed by specific biochemical tests on amniotic* fluid cells obtained by amniocentesis*. Pre-implantation* diagnosis from a single cell biopsy* taken from embryos generated by IVF* procedures is being studied; it will make it possible to limit embryo transfer to normal embryos, thus avoiding later antenatal diagnosis and possible termination of pregnancy.

teratogenesis: the processes leading to the development of structural or metabolic abnormalities in a fetus. These can be genetically determined or caused by environmental factors, such as maternal diseases, irradiation, drugs ingested in pregnancy or disorders of the placental circulation in multiple* pregnancies. Both genetic and environmental causes can together be operative in any one case.

teratozoospermia: semen* containing a high proportion of abnormally shaped spermatozoa* (i.e. abnormal sperm morphology*). According to the WHO* definition, teratozoopermia is a semen sample with less than 30% normal forms. The strict* criteria of Kruger regard semen with less than 4% normal forms as infertile. Absolute teratozoopermia occurs in globozoospermia* (in which the spermatozoa cannot fertilize because of failure of the development of the acrosome*) and in the immotile* cilia syndrome (no sperm motility due to abnormally developed tails).

TESA (Fig. 24): testicular sperm aspiration, usually carried out for ICSI* in irreversible obstructive* azoospermia where PESA* has been unsuccessful. Spermatozoa* are aspirated from the testis* by a fine needle under local or general anaesthesia. When sperm production is impaired (e.g. in primary testicular* failure), TESA is unlikely to be successful, and TESE (testicular sperm extraction from a biopsy*) is then used. (See also epididymal sperm aspiration.)

TESE: see testicular sperm extraction.

testicle (Fig. 15): anatomical term, describing the testis* with its ducts, including the epididymis* and scrotal* portion of the vas* deferens, its various coverings which include the spermatic fascia and the tunica* vaginalis, as well as the testicular blood vessels, lymphatics, nerves and cremaster muscle.

testicular biopsy: removal of a small amount of tissue from the testis* for diagnosis (e.g. infertility, suspected cancer) or treatment (e.g. TESE*). Biopsy can be performed by needle aspiration or by an open technique through a small scrotal* incision (the 'window technique') under local or general anaesthesia. An open biopsy provides more tissue for assessment.

Small, solitary (3 mm diameter) biopsies of each testis are usually adequate for histological assessment of sperm production, but in primary testicular* failure, the changes in the testes are often patchy and therefore multiple separate biopsies are required in the hope of detecting any minute sperm-containing foci. Precancerous changes (see carcinoma *in situ*) are sometimes found in biopsies obtained from infertile men: it is therefore advisable to request histological examination of at least one biopsy from each testis when a first TESE*/ICSI* treatment cycle is undertaken.

testicular failure: inability of the testis* to function normally. Both functions of the testis, the production of spermatozoa* and the secretion of testosterone*, may be affected.

Primary testicular failure may be congenital (e.g. Klinefelter's* syndrome, somatic chromosome* abnormalities), or due to undescended* testes, bilateral torsion, radiotherapy or mumps orchitis*. The clinical features include azoospermia* or severe oligospermia*, small testes and raised serum FSH* concentrations. Many patients have hypogonadism*. The infertility is usually incurable, but spermatozoa may be obtained by TESE* as there are minute patchy foci of sperm production in about 50% of patients. These can then be used for ICSI*. It is advisable in these cases to arrange genetic testing and counselling, in order to prevent the transmission of potentially undesirable genetic conditions. Symptoms of hypogonadism can be treated by testosterone administration, but this should be withheld until fertility treatment is completed as it may interfere with sperm production.

Secondary testicular failure is due to lack of gonadotrophin* hormone secretion by the pituitary* gland, and is usually referred to as hypogonadotrophic* hypogonadism. It is caused by pituitary or hypothalamic* disorders (tumours, meningitis, Kallmann's* syndrome). Patients may present with delayed puberty*, hypogonadism* or infertility*, all of which are cured by gonadotrophin* therapy.

testicular feminization syndrome (androgen insensitivity): in this syndrome, the individual has a 46 XY karyotype* and produces testosterone* which is inactive due to various abnormalities of the androgen* receptors in the developing fetal reproductive system. There is a vagina which ends as a blind pouch. The cervix, uterus, tubes and ovaries are absent. There is marked breast enlargement at puberty* and little pubic or axillary hair growth. The testes* remain in the pelvis or inguinal canal with an increased risk of malignancy. Their removal is recommended for this reason. Affected individuals are usually brought up as females and treatment with oestrogens may be recommended. (See also hermaphroditism.)

testicular obstruction: see azoospermia*, obstructive* azoospermia.

testicular sperm extraction (TESE) (Fig. 24): the extraction of spermatozoa* for ICSI* by testicular* biopsy. This is performed in men with azoospermia* due to primary testicular* failure or irreversible obstruction*, when MESA*, PESA* or TESA* have been unsuccessful. Local or general anaesthesia is employed. The testicular tissue is teased apart in the laboratory and examined by microscope; if obtained from men with obstructive azoospermia, spermatozoa, often with rudimentary activity, are readily identified. In primary testicular failure, the embryologist may have to search for many hours to find any spermatozoa which are usually very scanty and immotile.

testis (Fig. 25): the male gonad*, responsible for sexual development and fertility. Development of the testes is induced by the testis determining factor (TDF), located on the Y* chromosome. In the embryo, the testicular Leydig* cells secrete androgens* which promote development of the internal sperm conducting channels and the external genitalia (scrotum* and penis*). At puberty*, gonadotrophins*, secreted by the pituitary* gland, stimulate the testes to produce testosterone*,

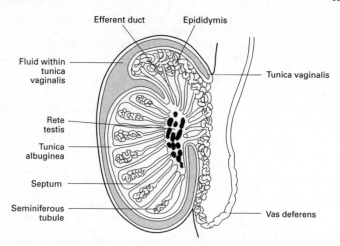

Fig. **25**. The Testis.

which, in turn, stimulates the development of the secondary sexual* characteristics and the initiation of spermatogenesis*.

There are two testes which descend into their separate compartments in the scrotum*. They are surrounded by the fluid-filled tunica* vaginalis which, if it persists in adult life, may predispose to inguinal hernia. The adult testis is oval, 4.5 to 5 cm long, and enclosed in the tough tunica* albuginea covering which thickens posteriorly to form the mediastinum. Fibrous septa extend between the mediastinum and the tunica albuginea to divide each testis into 200 to 400 compartments, each enclosing 1 to 4 convoluted seminiferous* tubules about 60 cm long. The tubules straighten, converge and amalgamate to become the rete* testis, a network of wide channels within the mediastinum from which 12 to 20 efferent ducts pierce the tunica albuginea and convey spermatozoa to the head (caput) of the epididymis*. (See also orchitis.)

testosterone: the principal male sex hormone*. Testosterone is an androgen*, derived from the cholesterol molecule, and therefore is a steroid* hormone. In adult males, about 90% of testosterone is produced by the Leydig* cells of the testes in response to pituitary gonadotrophins*, and about 10% is produced by the adrenal* glands.

Testosterone is responsible for the development and maintenance of the male reproductive system and the secondary sexual* characteristics. Spermatogenesis* requires a high local testosterone concentration within the testes. Deficiency of testosterone leads to hypogonadism* and is usually caused by testicular disorders, such as Klinefelter's* syndome or cryptorchism*. It may also be secondary to pituitary* deficiency. The peak testosterone level is reached at the age of 16 to 20 years, after which there is a gradual decline, but there is no evidence of a sudden drop or a male menopause*.

Proven testosterone deficiency may be treated by hormone* replacement therapy with depot injections, tablets or skin patches. In women, raised testosterone concentrations may occur in polycystic* ovarian syndrome, where there are virilizing changes (see hyperandrogenism). After the menopause*, testosterone may be administered to women, together with HRT*, to improve libido*.

thalassaemia: the commonest of the haemoglobinopathies* with a wide distribution in Africa, Asia, the Middle East and Mediterranean countries. The condition is genetically determined and is characterized by a reduction or lack of production of either the α or the β chain of haemoglobin. In homozygotes*, the red blood cells with the abnormal haemoglobin cannot function normally and disintegrate rapidly (haemolysis), resulting in severe anaemia and sometimes death. A fetus homozygous* for the severe form of α* thalassaemia is not viable. Those homozygous for β* thalassaemia have severe anaemia and die by their early twenties unless treated with repeated blood transfusions.

Many thalassaemia sufferers are now entering adult life and some of them may have a variety of endocrine* abnormalities due to the excess accumulation of iron (following many blood transfusions) in some of their ductless glands. Heterozygotes* are carriers; they may suffer mild anaemia. Female carriers should be identified by the antenatal screening* of those at risk. If the partner is also found to be a carrier, antenatal diagnosis can be performed on the fetus.

thalidomide: a drug first introduced in Germany in 1956 and widely used for sedation and treatment of nausea in early pregnancy. By 1961 it was linked to the appearance of severe fetal malformations if taken in the first trimester* of pregnancy. The most severe of the malformations were limb reduction abnormalities affecting both upper and lower limbs. Other abnormalities included malformations of the heart, ears, eyes and central nervous system. Thalidomide induced abnormalities in over 8000 babies born in 28 countries. One significance of the thalidomide tragedy was that it was the first realization that a non-toxic drug administered to a pregnant women could have severe teratogenic* effects.

theca cells: ovarian* interstitial cells which develop concentrically around the basement membrane of the follicle*. The layer adjacent to the basement membrane is the theca* interna and the outer layer is the theca* externa. Nerves and blood vessels are present in the theca but do not cross the basement membrane into the interior of the follicle. The theca interna cells secrete steroids*, particularly androgens*, which traverse the basement membrane for conversion to oestrogen* by the granulosa* cells.

theca externa: see theca cells.

theca interna: see theca cells.

theca lutein cells: see luteal cells.

threatened miscarriage: painless bleeding in early pregnancy, which may settle with normal continuation of the pregnancy or progress and be accompanied by pain to become an inevitable miscarriage*. First trimester* bleeding may also indicate an extra-uterine* pregnancy or a hydatidiform* mole; an ultrasound* scan can be performed to distinguish between these conditions.

In the presence of a viable fetus on the scan, the bleeding is thought to be either from the decidua* or an absorbing second gestational sac. Reassurance that most pregnancies with a viable fetus go to term is the mainstay of management. The administration of progesterone* or hCG* has been found to be ineffective and is no longer practiced. (See also abortion/miscarriage and early pregnancy loss.)

thrombosis: the occurrence of a blood clot in a blood vessel. Arterial thrombosis is usually associated with pathological changes in the wall of an artery* and causes acute symptoms by obstructing the circulation in the organ distal to the point of thrombosis, e.g. cerebral thrombosis (stroke) and coronary thrombosis. Venous thrombosis generally occurs in the veins of the legs or pelvis and may be associated with venous stasis due to immobilization (e.g. bed rest after childbirth or operations) or with abnormal changes of factors involved in the blood clotting mechanism.

An embolus* may result from the breaking off of part of an intravascular blood clot which is then transported by the blood stream to a distant site. Early diagnosis of thrombosis is essential and treatment with anticoagulants (heparin or warfarin) necessary for several months. Prophylactic heparin therapy for subsequent high risk activities (e.g. future pregnancies, surgery etc.) is recommended. (See also embolism.)

thrush: see *Candida albicans*, moniliasis.

thyroid: a large endocrine* gland, sited in front of and on both sides of the trachea in the neck. Stimulation of the thyroid gland by pituitary* thyrotrophic hormone (TSH) causes it to secrete its own hormones, mainly T4 (thyroxine), and T3 (tri-iodo thyronine) which influence metabolic processes throughout the body. TSH production is itself under the control of the hypothalamic* TSH-releasing hormone. The thyroid gland also secretes calcitonin which inhibits bone resorption. Oestrogens* and testosterone* stimulate calcitonin secretion and levels fall in postmenopausal women.

Congenital thyroid deficiency causes cretinism while thyroid deficiency in later life causes myxoedema*. Overactivity of the thyroid gland causes thyrotoxicosis* and, sometimes, Graves' disease (exophthalmic goitre). (See hyperthyroidism, hypothyroidism.)

thyrotoxicosis: see hyperthyroidism.

timed intercourse: intercourse undertaken or avoided at the fertile time of the cycle (see fertile period). Many women are aware of their fertile period as a result of changes in their cervical mucus and vaginal fluid. Incorrect timing of intercourse in the cycle can be a cause of subfertility. High technology methods of timing ovulation*, such as serial ultrasound* scans or biochemical markers, are usually reserved for timing of artificial* insemination, but do-it-yourself kits are now available to allow women to identify their own LH* surge in order to enhance or avoid their chances of conception.

toxaemia: see pre-eclampsia.

toxoplasmosis: infection caused by *Toxoplasma gondii*. This is an intracellular protozoon parasite which infects a wide range of animal species and a large proportion of the human population, in addition to its natural host, the cat. Only 10 to 20% of toxoplasma infections cause symptoms which include swollen lymph glands, fever, malaise and sore throat. Following the initial infection, the parasite establishes a latent infection in the form of cysts in various tissues, including muscle and brain.

Transmission from mother to fetus can result from primary infections occurring at any time from 6 to 8 weeks before conception until the third trimester* of pregnancy. The frequency of transmission increases during the course of the pregnancy, from 10 to 25% in the first trimester to 70 to 90% in the third, but the effects of transmission on the fetus are most severe in the first trimester and least severe in the third. Affected infants suffer from blindness and mental retardation. Infection can be prevented by avoidance of cats, raw or undercooked meat and incompletely washed vegetables. Treatment of infected mothers with pyrimethanine and spiramycin has been shown to be effective in preventing transmission to the fetus.

transcription: the production of a genetic template (messenger RNA*) from DNA*, used by the cell* for the production of proteins*.

transgenic: a transgenic organism is one that has had its genetic material (DNA*) altered through genetic engineering so that it contains one or more genes* from another species in all of its cells*. At present, the transgenic alteration of humans is illegal in the UK. Such alteration is also known as germline gene therapy (see gene therapy). However, the creation of transgenic micro-organisms, fungi, plants and animals is becoming increasingly common. For example, transgenic crops which are more resistant to diseases are being produced, while research has enabled transgenic sheep to produce therapeutic human proteins in their milk.

translocation: a type of mutation* in which a whole chromosome* or part of one is attached to another chromosome or moves to a different place within the same chromosome. Translocations vary in their clinical significance. One form of Down's* syndrome is the result of a translocation (see Robertsonian translocation).

treponema pallidum: the causative agent of syphilis, a member of a large group of organisms known as spirochaetes. (See syphilis.)

trial: a scientific investigation where there is some measure of design (randomized trial, cross-over trial, clinical trial) and which can be subjected to statistical* analysis. Trials are frequently employed in medicine to assess the effectiveness of a treatment or intervention or to compare two or more different treatments.

trichomonas: a wide-spread sexually* transmitted disease, caused by a protozoan organism, *Trichomonas vaginalis*. It causes inflammation of the vulva* and vagina* with a frothy, green or yellow malodorous discharge. Although transmitted by men, it rarely causes symptoms in males. Treatment is with metronidazole tablets which should be prescribed for both partners to avoid re-infection.

trimester: time span of three months. Pregnancy is nominally subdivided into the first trimester (up to 13 weeks), the second trimester (up to the 26th week) and the third trimester (from the 27th week until term).

triplets: three babies delivered at the same birth. (See multiple pregnancy.)

triploidy: a form of polyploidy* in which a cell's nucleus* contains three times the haploid* complement. Most triploid embryos miscarry. Occasionally they are associated with the formation of a hydatidiform* mole.

In IVF*, a triploid embryo is normally recognized by the presence of three pronuclei*. A gynogenetic triploid embryo has two pronuclei contributed by the oocyte* (usually because of failure of extrusion of the second polar* body) and has been fertilized by a single spermatozoon. More commonly, *in vitro*, triploidy results from the simultaneous fertilization of one oocyte by two spermatozoa. Triploid embryos are not used for embryo* transfer.

trisomy: abnormal genetic constitution in which there are three copies of one particular chromosome. The commonest trisomy in humans is Down's* syndrome, trisomy 21. Most fetuses with other trisomies miscarry, e.g. Edwards' syndrome (trisomy 18) and Patau syndrome (trisomy 13): if born alive, they have multiple abnormalities and die in childhood. (See also monosomy, Down's syndrome.)

trophectoderm (*syn.* trophoblast): the outer single-cell layer of the blastocyst*. The trophectoderm cells are linked by tight junctions. All metabolic processes in the blastocele* are therefore regulated since all components must pass through or be secreted by the trophectoderm cells. The internal environment surrounding the inner* cell mass (which will form the fetus) is thereby strictly controlled.

After hatching*, the trophectoderm makes the initial contact with the endometrial* cells, leading to implantation*. The trophectoderm secretes human* chorionic gonadotrophin (hCG) in large amounts, the presence of which forms the basis of pregnancy* tests. The trophectoderm forms the extra-embryonic membranes, including the chorion* from which the placenta* eventually develops. (See also blastocyst, chorion.)

tubal insufflation test: a test, also known as the Rubin test after its originator, performed to ascertain the patency of the Fallopian* tubes by the transcervical passage of carbon* dioxide gas; manometric recordings of pressure changes in the tubes are made during the insufflation. The test can be misleading and has now been replaced by other investigations such as hystero-salpingography*, laparoscopy*, salpingoscopy* and falloposcopy* which are more reliable and informative.

tubal pregnancy: see extra-uterine/ectopic pregnancy.

tube: see Fallopian tube.

tuberculosis: a chronic infection caused by *Mycobacterium tuberculosis*. Genital tuberculosis affects primarily the Fallopian* tubes with secondary spread to the endometrium*. It is usually blood-borne from a primary focus in the lungs, lymph glands, urinary tract or bones. Affected tubes may appear almost normal, may be swollen and reddened, or may be enlarged as bilateral pyosalpinges*.

Infection causes infertility and there is tubal occlusion in more than 50% of affected patients. Treatment is with long-term triple antibiotic therapy. Apart from infertility, the infection may cause no other symptoms or there may be menstrual disturbances including menorrhagia* and amenorrhoea*.

Genital tuberculosis tends to occur in women who have their primary focus after the menarche. In the UK, with a reduced incidence of pulmonary tuberculosis and BCG vaccination of young girls, genital tuberculosis is rare and no longer a significant cause of infertility. In countries where the incidence of pulmonary tuberculosis is high, genital tuberculosis remains a frequent cause of infertility, difficult to treat. IVF* is the treatment of choice, although the success rate is lower than average in this condition.

In men, genital tract infection with tuberculosis leads to tuberculous epididymitis* or scarring of the vas* deferens, causing obstructive* azoospermia*.

tubo-ovarian abscess: a life-threatening complication of pelvic* inflammatory disease, causing distension with pus of the Fallopian* tube(s) and adherent ovary. In acute cases there is a raised temperature, abdominal pain and general malaise. Treatment is by surgical drainage and antibiotics. Rupture causes peritonitis which can be fatal.

Tubo-ovarian cysts, which may represent a final, burned-out stage of a tubo-ovarian abscess, are usually asymptomatic and discovered on pelvic examination. Infertility occurs in both the acute and chronic stages due to tubal occlusion and interference with normal ovulation.

TUDOR: transvaginal ultrasound* directed oocyte retrieval, used for IVF*. See oocyte collection.

tunica albuginea: term used to describe a membrane which encloses an organ. In women, this is the layer of connective tisue immediately beneath the germinal* epithelium of the ovary*. In men, the tunica albuginea is the fibrous outer layer of the testis. (See testis.)

tunica vaginalis (Fig. 25): the outer part of the capsule which encloses the testis* and its tunica* albuginea. The tunica vaginalis, which is developmentally continuous with the peritoneal* cavity, has two layers enclosing a small amount of serous fluid. This permits movement of the testis in the scrotum*. (See testis.)

Turner's syndrome: a congenital* disorder affecting the approximately one in 3000 females who have one X chromosome* missing, i.e. are 45/XO. As two complete and normal X chromosomes are needed for normal ovarian* development, affected females have failure of ovarian function. They exhibit sexual infantilism and short stature and may have webbing of the neck, valgus deformity of the elbows, and coarctation (narrowing) of the aorta. In adolescence*, there is no breast development, no growth of pubic or axillary hair and usually no onset of menstruation*. Mental development is normal. There is a raised serum FSH* concentration and on laparoscopy* small, fibrous 'streak' ovaries are seen; the uterus and tubes are present, but small.

The ovarian dysgenesis is probably due to rapid and early regression of follicles*, before the menarche*, i.e. a form of premature* ovarian failure, rather than to the congenital absence of oocytes*. This explains the occasional occurrence of menstruation and, very rarely, pregnancy. Treatment with cyclical hormone* replacement therapy (usually a combined oral contraceptive pill) is started in adolescence, and pregnancies have been achieved with egg* donation. (See also gonadal dysgenesis, monosomy.)

twins: two babies delivered at the same birth. (See multiple pregnancy.)

U

ultrasound/ultrasonography: the use of high frequency sound waves to identify bodily structures. The waves are directed as a beam by a hand held transducer and their echoes, which are bounced off the organ under examination, are shown as electric images on a monitor screen. In gynaecology, both abdominal and vaginal transducers are used. Originally introduced for the visualization of a fetus or ovarian cysts*, ultrasound techniques have advanced rapidly to become the most widely used non-invasive method of investigation of normal and abnormal structures.

Ultrasound is used for the early diagnosis of pregnancy, monitoring of embryonic and fetal growth and wellbeing, placental localization and many other purposes. In cases of miscarriage*, it is used to determine whether a pregnancy is viable and whether a miscarriage, if it has occurred, is complete or incomplete.

In reproductive medicine, ultrasound is used to examine the uterus* for congenital abnormalities or for the presence of fibroids* and to measure the thickness of the endometrium*. The ovaries are examined for normal follicular* development and for the presence of ovarian cysts* or polycystic* ovarian syndrome. Ovarian* stimulation is monitored with ultrasound, and oocyte* collection for IVF* is performed under ultrasound guidance.

In men, scrotal* ultrasound may be used for the detection of varicoceles*, spermatoceles* or testicular tumours. Transrectal ultrasound can be used to identify dilatation of the seminal* vesicles when ejaculatory duct obstruction is suspected and is also used for the diagnosis of prostate* disorders, including cancer. (See also Doppler.)

umbilical cord: the thick structure, resembling a spirally twisted rope, which connects the fetus* to the placenta*. The cord, which is variable in length, but usually more than 55 cm long at term, consists of a jelly-like substance which contains the single umbilical vein and the two umbilical arteries. Nutrients, oxygen, hormones and other substances are delivered to the fetus via the umbilical vein while by-products of metabolism and carbon dioxide are excreted to the placenta, and hence the maternal circulation, via the arteries.

Interference to the blood flow through the umbilical vessels can be caused by knots in the cord, twisting of the cord around the fetal neck or prolapse and compression of the cord during labour, causing fetal anoxia. For antenatal diagnosis, fetal blood sampling (e.g. in order to establish the fetal karyotype*) can be performed by ultrasound*-guided aspiration of blood from cord vessels.

undescended testes (cryptorchidism): a developmental abnormality, occurring in 1 to 3% of male infants, when one or both testes* fail to migrate properly from their site of formation on the posterior abdominal wall of the embryo, through the inguinal canal, into the scrotum*. Testes may be incompletely or maldescended if arrested along this path, often inside the inguinal canal, in association with a hernia. Ectopic testes have strayed from this path and may be under the skin of the groin or thigh.

Leydig* cell function and testosterone* secretion are normal, and so even children with bilateral cryptorchidism mature normally. There is a risk of infertility, due to impaired spermatogenesis*, and of testicular cancer, torsion and trauma. Treatment may be tried in the first year of life with the administration of GnRH* or hCG*; if this is not successful, the testis should be fixed in the scrotum by the operation of orchidopexy by the age of 2 years. In adults, any unexplained absent testis is assumed to be undescended and so surgical exploration is undertaken to relocate or remove an undescended testis to prevent the development of malignancy.

Retractile testes are sensitive with highly active spermatic* cord (cremaster) muscles which draw them into the groin, but careful examination reveals they are normally descended when the patient is relaxed and no treatment is necessary.

unexplained infertility: infertility* for which no cause is found after full investigation of both partners. Routine tests will include semen analysis*, a post-coital test*, search for evidence of ovulation* and determination of tubal status by hysterosalpingography* or laparoscopy*. If these do not determine a definite cause, further tests may be performed to detect antisperm* antibodies or sperm* dysfunction. Many cases of unexplained infertility are probably the result of minor degrees of impairment of ovulation*, sperm function or endometrial* development for which no adequate tests exist at present.

Treatment of unexplained infertility includes attempts to improve the quality of ovulation by three to four courses of clomiphene* citrate, ovarian* stimulation with gonadotrophins*, followed by intra-uterine* insemination or the use of IVF*. One of the advantages of treatment with IVF is that it gives the opportunity of determining whether fertilization* does or does not occur in a particular couple.

uniovular twins: see monozygotic twins.

urethra: the hollow tube through which urine is expelled from the bladder. In women, the urethra terminates at the external urinary meatus in the introitus* just above the vaginal* orifice. The female urethra is short (2 to 4 cm) and this is one reason why ascending infections have ready access to the bladder, causing cystitis*. The male urethra is about 25 cm long and therefore urinary infections are rare in young men.

utero–tubal junction (Fig. 26): the place where the Fallopian* tube enters the uterine* cavity. A sphincter-like mechanism is present at the junction and is under hormonal* control, so that the junction is virtually closed during menstruation* (preventing retrograde menstruation) and relaxed at midcycle.

The utero–tubal junction has an important role in the transport of spermatozoa* through the genital tract and in the precise timing of the entry of the embryo* into the uterine cavity.

The utero–tubal junction is one of the common sites of tubal occlusion which is usually due to preceding infection, but may also be due to polyps or mucus plugs. Such obstructions are diagnosed by hystero-salpingography*, laparoscopy* or fallopscopy* and are treatable by balloon catheterization or tubal microsurgery*. Conception failure after such procedures is an important indication for IVF*.

uterus (Fig. 26): the thick-walled, potentially hollow organ situated in the female pelvis, shaped like an inverted pear, 8–9 cm long, 6 cm wide and 4 cm thick in the non-pregnant adult. It is subdivided into the body (corpus), isthmus and cervix*. The Fallopian* tubes open into the upper part of the body (the fundus) at the uterine angles (cornua) and via the uterine cavity, communicate with the vagina through the cervical canal.

The outer surface of the uterus (except where the bladder is attached anteriorly, and the supporting ligaments laterally) is covered by peritoneum (the serosa). The bulk of the uterus consists of the myometrium*, specialized bundles of non-striated (smooth) muscle, capable of enormous stretching and growth in pregnancy, contraction and retraction in labour and, by virtue of its criss-cross muscle fibre arrangement, arrest of bleeding after the separation of the placenta*. Internally, the uterine cavity has a highly specialized lining, the endometrium*, which undergoes cyclical changes in response to the ovarian* hormones*, develops into the decidua* if conception* has occurred, or is shed (menstruation*) if there has been no conception.

The endometrium reacts to disturbances of the ovarian hormones (see menstrual disorders) and, like any other mucous membrane, can produce polyps* and undergo hyperplastic* or malignant changes. The myometrium is a frequent site of fibroids* and adenomyosis*. Congenital abnormalities of the uterus are mostly due

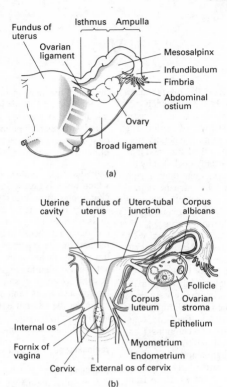

Fig. **26**. Uterus, Fallopian tube and ovary. Posterior view of the organs (a) intact, (b) sectioned.

to fusion failures of the Müllerian* ducts: they rarely cause infertility but may be associated with miscarriages*, especially in the second trimester* of pregnancy.

Retroversion* of the uterus is common, but only occasionally relevant to infertility. Congenital absence of the uterus (Rokitansky–Kuester–Mayer syndrome) is rare. In this syndrome there is normal ovarian function. The condition, like hysterectomy* in a young woman, may be an indication for surrogacy*, using the affected woman's own oocytes*. (See also cervix, myometrium, endometrium, men-struation, utero–tubal junction, utriculoplasty.)

utriculoplasty: non-specific name given to reconstructive operations on the uterus for the correction of fusion failures (partial or complete) of the Müllerian* ducts. Formerly performed by open surgery (see Strassman* operation), these operations are now mostly performed through the hystero-scope* with shorter hospitalization, less post-operative pain and no risk of adhesion formation. They are only indicated in women with recurrent* miscarriages and no living child.

V

vagina (*lit.* sheath): the elastic canal, approximately 10 cm long, which passes from the vulva* into the pelvis in an upward and backward direction. The entrance to the vagina is generally closed by apposition of the labia* and may or may not be partially occluded by the hymen*. At its upper end it terminates blindly as a vault into which the vaginal part of the cervix* projects; the areas surrounding this are the anterior, posterior and two lateral fornices*.

The vagina has a muscular wall, enclosed in an elastic sheath, and is capable of enormous dilatation, constituting the lower end of the birth canal. After delivery there is usually some laxity in these tissues. Internally it is lined by a thin stratified epithelium* which has no secretory function. The vaginal fluid consists of secretions from the cervical glands and transudation of fluid from the vaginal epithelium. This fluid is acidic, particularly when the ovarian* homones* are active, i.e. from puberty* to the menopause*, thus providing at least some protection against ascending infections. (See also vaginitis, vaginosis, vaginismus.)

vaginal fornix: see fornix.

vaginismus: an involuntary spasm of the muscles surrounding the vaginal entrance when attempts are made to introduce the penis, examining finger, or any other object into the vagina. Vaginismus may affect 1 in 200 women and is a common cause of non-consummation, sexual dysfunction, dyspareunia and infertility. The patient may find it difficult to admit to it in the history taking and the condition is then diagnosed either during the routine pelvic examination or during the performance of a post-coital* test.

Vaginismus is a psychosomatic disorder, induced by fear of penetration and deep anxiety. It may be related to sexual abuse in childhood or other forms of childhood/adolescent trauma and it may induce impotence* in a newly married, sexually inexperienced partner. Treatment is mainly by psychotherapy and behavioural therapy initiated by Masters and Johnson, combined with teaching patients about their own anatomy and inducing them to explore this by self-examination.

vaginitis: inflammation of the vagina* which usually presents with a discharge and irritation. The commonest sexually transmitted cause of vaginitis is trichomoniasis*. Candidiasis* is common in diabetics and may occur in patients on oral contraceptive pills and those treated with prolonged courses of antibiotics. 'Senile' vaginitis occurs in post-menopausal* women and is due to lack of oestrogens* and their protective effect on the vaginal epithelium. Any abnormal discharge should be investigated by microscopy and bacteriology.

vaginosis: see bacterial vaginosis.

vanishing fetus: the death of a fetus in a multiple pregnancy, diagnosed by ultrasound*. See multiple pregnancy.

varicella zoster virus (chickenpox): this virus infection is common in childhood, usually mild, with a typical vesicular rash. Shingles (herpes zoster) results from reactivation of the virus that has remained latent in the body after the first infection.

Chickenpox in pregnancy can have grave consequences for both the mother and the fetus. In pregnant women, it can become a serious and even fatal disease; those who deteriorate, particularly with the onset of respiratory symptoms, require hospitalization and urgent treatment. Maternal infection in the first half of pregnancy carries up to a 4% chance of fetal abnormalities, which include microcephaly and skin and muscle scarring. Infection around the time of delivery signals a risk of severe infection in the infant. Shingles does not carry significant risks for the mother or fetus.

Effective drug therapy for chickenpox exists, and prophylactic treatment with immune globulin has also been shown to have some protective effect if given within 10 days of exposure to chickenpox.

varicocele: an abnormal accumulation of dilated (varicose) veins* of the pampiniform plexus of the spermatic* cord. Varicoceles occur in 1 in 5 men, predominantly on the left side, but are often bilateral. They are caused by abnormal reflux of blood due to incompetence of the spermatic veins which drain the testis*.

The increased blood flow into the scrotum* raises the temperature of both testes, leading to a deterioration in sperm* production. Varicoceles occur in 1 in 3 infertile men, and can be treated by surgical ligation of the internal spermatic veins or by obliteration through the insertion of coils into the incompetent veins. After such procedures, the sperm count may rise and spontaneous pregnancy may occur in up to 50% of couples within 2 years. However, many andrologists* are not convinced that varicoceles are an important cause of male infertility because they are also common in fertile men.

vas deferens (Fig. 15): the duct which transports spermatozoa* from the epididymis* to the accessory* glands at the base of the bladder which secrete the seminal* plasma. The vas arises from the tail of the epididymis* at the lower pole of the testis* and passes with the spermatic* cord, through the inguinal canal, into the abdominal cavity towards the base of the bladder. It forms an ampulla above the prostate* gland, which acts as a reservoir for spermatozoa, and is joined by the duct of the seminal* vesicle; it then meets its fellow at the midline to form the paired ejaculatory* ducts which penetrate the prostate and open into the urethra*. The vas is about 30 cm long, and has a narrow lumen and a thick muscular coat to propel the spermatozoa.

Bilateral congenital absence of the vas (BCAV) occurs in about 1 in 1000 men and is a cause of obstructive* azoospermia. The vas can be obstructed by scarring following gonorrhoea* or tuberculosis*, or inadvertently during surgical repair of an inguinal hernia. Male sterilization* is carried out by dividing both vasa (see vasectomy).

vasectomy: a male sterilization* operation involving the division of both vasa (see vas deferens). The operation is usually performed above the testis*, in the scrotum*, under local anaesthesia. It is not effective immediately since spermatozoa are stored in the ampulla of the vas and in the seminal* vesicles and about 12 ejaculations are required to empty them. Unprotected intercourse is deemed safe after two consecutive semen* samples, examined at 12 and 16 weeks after surgery, are found to be clear of spermatozoa. Spontaneous recanalization can occur in 1 in 2500 cases up to many years later, and therefore patients must be warned that the operation is not 100% effective. Following vasectomy, sexual function, spermatogenesis* and hormone* production remain normal. (See vasectomy reversal.)

vasectomy reversal: this is technically feasible by surgical anastomosis* with about a 90% chance of restoring spermatozoa* to the semen*. However, even when successful, the return of fertility is reduced to about 40 to 50% due to the appearance of antisperm* antibodies. Vasectomy* should therefore be considered irreversible and prior counselling of both partners is advisable. This is particularly important as requests for vasectomy may sometimes be associated with sexual or marital problems. (See vasectomy, vaso-vasostomy.)

vasogram: a radiological examination of the vas* deferens, after injection of a radio-opaque dye into its lumen. Patency is shown by the presence of dye in the bladder, whilst in cases of obstruction the site of the block may be demonstrated. Vasography is usually performed before epididymo*-vasostomy or vaso*-vasostomy are undertaken in the treatment of obstructive* azoospermia.

vaso-epididymostomy: see epididymo-vasostomy.

vaso-vasostomy: anastomosis* to rejoin the divided vas* deferens after excision of a block in obstructive* azoospermia, or for the reversal* of vasectomy*. Microsurgical* techniques are usually employed and the operation is usually performed under general anaesthesia.

vein: blood vessel which returns blood to the heart from the various structures and organs of the body. Veins have valves to prevent reverse (reflux) flow, thereby assisting in the return of blood to the heart.

venereal disease: disease transmitted by sexual contact. The statutory diseases, requiring notification, are syphilis*, gonorrhoea* and chancroid. (See sexually transmitted disease.)

Verres needle: a specially adapted needle used in laparoscopy* for the insufflation of the peritoneal cavity with carbon dioxide gas. The needle has a sharp pointed outer barrel to pierce the abdominal wall and a blunt inner cannula to pierce the peritoneum and avoid damage to bowel.

vestibule: see introitus.

villi: see chorionic villi.

virus: viruses infect every form of life, from bacteria to humans. They are a hugely diverse group of organisms whose only common features are their small size (all but the largest family, pox viruses, are too small to be seen using light microscopy) and their inability to replicate their genetic material without the 'machinery' present in the cells they infect.
  Viruses affect reproductive medicine in three ways. They are a rare cause of infertility, for example the mumps* virus which may cause testicular atrophy following mumps orchitis*. They can cause stillbirth* or fetal abnormalities through intrauterine infections, for example rubella* virus, cytomegalovirus* and human* immunodeficiency virus (HIV). Finally, they can cause risks to health care workers involved in reproductive medicine, for example the human* immunodeficiency virus and hepatitis* viruses B and C.

virilization: see hyperandrogenism.

viscosity: a measure of the fluidity of a liquid. Semen* coagulates immediately after ejaculation*, then usually liquifies within 20 to 60 minutes. Prostatitis* may lead to increased and prolonged viscosity of the seminal* fluid, but the effect of this on sperm function is uncertain.

vitelline membrane: see oolemma.

vitrification: method of cryopreservation* which uses high concentrations of cryoprotectants* and rapid cooling to produce a 'glass', thereby avoiding problems of crystal formation. This method is not usually used in human oocyte or embryo cryopreservation because of the potentially toxic effect of the high concentrations of cryoprotectants required.

Voluntary Licensing Authority (VLA): body set up jointly by the Medical Research Council and the Royal College of Obstetricians and Gynaecologists in 1985, following publication of the Warnock Report in 1984. The Warnock committee was set up by the UK Parliament in 1982 to inquire into human fertilization and embryology. One of its principal recommendations was that a new statutory licensing authority should be established to regulate certain types of infertility treatment and related research. The VLA, later known as the Interim* Licensing Authority, laid down a code of practice on research related to human fertilization and embryology and set up a system of visiting and licensing clinics in which IVF* and certain other procedures were undertaken. This work continued until the establishment of the Human* Fertilisation and Embryology Authority in 1991.

vulva (Fig. 27): the external part of the female genital tract, consisting of the area enclosed by the mons veneris, labia* majora and perineum* and including the labia minora, clitoris*, introitus* and vaginal orifice.

vulvitis: inflammation of the vulva*; this can be due to infections such as candidiasis* and herpes*, to chemical irritants such as detergents, soaps, bubble baths and sprays, or to some specific skin conditions such as eczema, psoriasis, lichen sclerosus and lichen planus. Vulvitis is also common in diabetics, and in postmenopausal women due to oestrogen* deficiency.

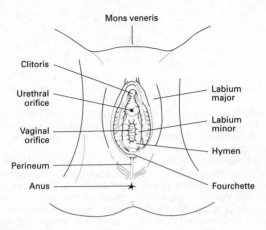

Fig. **27**. Vulva. The external female genitalia, including the introitus.

W

warts: see condylomata acuminata.

wedge resection: surgical procedure, involving the excision of a wedge-shaped part of the ovarian* cortex. The operation, employed in the treatment of polycystic* ovarian syndrome, was initially performed by open abdominal surgery and later through the laparoscope*. Laparoscopic ovarian wedge resection has been superseded by the use of ovarian diathermy or laser* vaporization.

Wolffian duct: embryonic structure from which the urinary tract is formed in both sexes. In the male, the body and tail of the epididymis*, the vas* deferens, seminal* vesicles and ejaculatory* ducts arise from the Wolffian ducts. Thus in congenital absence of the vas (see vas deferens) due to failure of Wolffian duct development, only the head of the epididymis is present. In the female, the Wolffian duct structures generally disappear or become rudimentary, but occasionally remnants persist, such as Gärtner's duct.

World Health Organisation (WHO): body set up in 1948 as the specialized agency of health of the United Nations. Its forerunner was the health section of the League of Nations between the two world wars. The League had some impact on women's health with the introduction of the international staging for cervical cancer.

The WHO, which is based in Geneva with posts around the world, has made outstanding contributions to health in the developing world, the most notable being the campaigns for the elimination of smallpox and malaria. The WHO also provides scientific and technical advice and sets international standards of normal values (e.g. semen*). In its Maternal and Child Health Division it has established 'Safe Motherhood' and 'Fertility Control' as its main objectives.

Other examples of its activities include the WHO Special Programme of Research Development and Research Training in Human Reproduction, the WHO Task Force on Prevention and Management of Infertility, and the publication of manuals on the examination of human semen and sperm–mucus interaction and on standardized investigation and diagnosis of the infertile couple. The WHO has also set up a collaborating centre for community control of hereditary diseases.

X

X chromosome: one of the two sex chromosomes*. The presence of two X chromosomes determines that an individual is female. The X chromosome carries a large number of genes* that play no role in sex determination. Disorders relating to these genes cause sex-linked abnormalities. (See chromosomes, sex chromosomes, sex determination, sex-linked abnormalities.)

X-linked genetic disorder: see sex-linked abnormalities.

XYY syndrome: the presence of two Y* chromosomes in a male, occurring in about 1 in 700 newborn males. Affected males are taller than average, but remain fertile. There is a higher than average incidence of mental retardation in these individuals and there is a certain amount of controversial evidence which suggests that they are more likely, at some time in their lives, to serve a custodial sentence for anti-social behaviour.

Y

Y chromosome: one of the two types of sex chromosomes*. The presence of a Y chromosome causes a fetus to develop as a male who thus has an XY karyotype*. The Y chromosome is the smallest chromosome in humans; apart from the sex determining factor, it carries few other genes*. (See also chromosomes, sex chromosomes, sex determination, sex-linked abnormalities.)

yolk sac: a very early embryonic structure, pear-shaped and about 5 mm wide by the end of the second month of pregnancy. It develops with the fetal membranes (see amnion and chorion) and is continuous with the embryonic gut. It probably has a role in the passage of nutrients to the early embryo but may be vestigial in humans. The yolk sac eventually shrinks and converts into a narrow solid band. When the proximal end of the sac persists, it is known as a Meckel's diverticulum of the ileum and can be associated with surgical complications. The yolk sac is one of the earliest embryonic organs that can be visualized by ultrasound*, around day 25 after conception.

Young's syndrome: a rare syndrome* in men, in which there is an association of obstructive* azoospermia with diseases of the lungs or sinuses (bronchiectasis, frequent respiratory infections, sinusitis). The aetiology remains uncertain, but mercury poisoning in childhood has been implicated and the incidence of this syndrome has declined, possibly due to the abolition of mercury-containing teething powders.

Z

Zoladex: see goserelin.

zona drilling: see assisted fertilization.

zona pellucida (Fig. 17): the gelatinous coat which encloses the oocyte*, separated from the oolemma* by the perivitelline* space and surrounded on its outer aspect by the cumulus* cells. The zona protects the oocyte* and early embryo and helps to prevent polyspermy* (penetration of the oocyte by more than one spermatozoon*: see zona reaction). To achieve fertilization*, the spermatozoon must bind to and penetrate the zona pellucida in order to reach the oocyte. After this, the zona* reaction prevents penetration of the oocyte by further spermatozoa.

The zona encloses the early embryo until it becomes a blastocyst*. The blastocyst has to escape from the zona pellucida before implantation* can occur (see hatching). Certain procedures in assisted* reproductive technology, such as prolonged culture or cryopreservation*, can cause hardening of the zona, and assisted* fertilization techniques such as zona drilling or partial* zona dissection (PZD) may be employed to facilitate hatching of the early embryo. (See also corona, cumulus, implantation.)

zona reaction: mechanism which prevents polyspermic* fertilization* by rendering the oocyte's* zona* pellucida impenetrable to all but the first fertilizing spermatozoon*. The zona reaction is mediated by release of cortical* granules from the oocyte as the fertilizing sperm penetrates it. The cortical granules contain enzymes* which interact with the inner surface of the zona pellucida, changing its structure and rendering it impassable to other spermatozoa. (See also zona pellucida, cortical granules.)

zygote: the fertilized oocyte*, normally with a diploid* chromosome complement and the presence of two pronuclei*. This is the first stage in the development of the embryo before cleavage* occurs.

Appendix 1

Abbreviations

This list refers to abbreviations used in this text. In every-day practice in reproductive medicine, some terms and procedures are generally referred to, and often better known, by their initials, e.g. DNA, IVF, ICSI, and have been listed thus in the text.

ACTH	adrenocorticotrophic hormone
AFP	alpha feto-protein
AI	artificial insemination
AID	artificial insemination with donor semen (*see* DI)
AIDS	acquired immunodeficiency syndrome
AIH	artificial insemination with husband's semen
ARIC	acrosome reaction with ionophore challenge
ART	assisted reproduction technology
AZF	azoospermia factor
β hCG	β human chorionic gonadotrophin
BBT	basal body temperature
BCAVD	bilateral congenital absence of the vas deferens
BP	blood pressure
BSO	bilateral salpingo-oophorectomy
BV	bacterial vaginosis
CASA	computer assisted sperm analysis
CAV	congenital absence of the vas deferens
CC	clomiphene citrate
CCR	cumulative conception rate
CIN	cervical intra-epithelial neoplasia
CMV	cytomegalovirus
CO_2	carbon dioxide
CT	computerized tomography (scan)
CPK	creatinine phosphokinase
CVS	chorionic villus sampling
	cardiovascular system
Cx	cervix
D & C	dilatation and curettage
DES	diethyl stilboestrol
DI	donor insemination
DIPI	direct intra-peritoneal insemination
DNA	deoxyribonucleic acid

E_1	œstrone
E_2	17 β œstradiol
E_3	œstriol
EGF	epidermal growth factor
ELISA	enzyme-linked immunosorbent assay
ERPC	evacuation of retained products of conception
ET	embryo transfer
FER	frozen embryo replacement
FISH	fluorescence *in situ* hybridization
FSH	follicle stimulating hormone
GIFT	gamete intrafallopian transfer
GnRH	gonadotrophin releasing hormone
hCG	human chorionic gonadotrophin
HFEA	Human Fertilisation and Embryology Authority
H-H	head to head sperm agglutination
HIV	human immunodeficiency virus
hMG	human menopausal gonadotrophin
HOS	hypo-osmotic swelling test
HPF	high power field
HPV	human papilloma virus
HRT	hormone replacement therapy
HSG	hysterosalpingogram
HSV	herpes simplex virus
H-T	head to tail sperm agglutination
IBT	immunobead test
ICM	inner cell mass
ICSI	intracytoplasmic sperm injection
Ig	immunoglobulin
IGF	insulin-like growth factor
ILA	Interim Licensing Authority
IMB	intermenstrual bleeding
IPI	intraperitoneal insemination
IU	international unit
IUCD	intra-uterine contraceptive device
IUD	intra-uterine death
IUI	intra-uterine insemination
IVF	*In vitro* fertilization
IVF-ET	*In vitro* fertilization and embryo transfer
LH	luteinizing hormone
LHD	lateral head displacement (of sperm when swimming)
LHRH	luteinizing hormone releasing hormone (=GnRH)
LSCS	lower segment caesarean section
LUF	luteinized unruptured follicle
MAR	mixed antiglobulin reaction

MESA	microsurgical epididymal sperm aspiration
MFT	male fertility test (semen analysis)
MRI	magnetic resonance imaging (scan)
MSU	midstream specimen of urine
NSU	non-specific urethritis
O_2	oxygen
OAT(S)	oligo-astheno-terato-zoospermia (syndrome)
OHSS	ovarian hyperstimulation syndrome
PAP	Papanicolaou (smear)
PCO	polycystic ovaries
PCOD	polycystic ovarian disease
PCOS	polycystic ovarian syndrome
PCR	polymerase chain reaction
PCT	post-coital test
PE	pre-eclampsia
PET	pre-eclamptic toxaemia
PESA	percutaneous epididymal sperm aspiration
PG	prostaglandin
PGD	pre-implantation genetic diagnosis
PGE	prostaglandin E
pH	a measure of acidity
PID	pelvic inflammatory disease
PKU	phenylketonuria
PMB	post-menopausal bleeding
PMS	pre-menstrual syndrome
PMT	pre-menstrual tension
PN	pronucleus
PNMR	perinatal mortality rate
POD	pouch of Douglas
POF	premature ovarian failure
POST	peritoneal oocyte and sperm transfer
PPH	post-partum haemorrhage
PROST	pronuclear stage transfer
PSA	prostate specific antigen
PZD	partial zona dissection
RETA	rete testis aspiration
Rh	rhesus (blood group)
RNA	ribonucleic acid
ROS	reactive oxygen species
RPC	retained products of conception
RU 486	mifepristone
SBK	spinnbarkeit
SCI	spinal cord injury
SCMC	sperm-cervical mucus contact test

SEM	scanning electron microscopy
SFA	seminal fluid analysis
SIFT	transvaginal intrafallopian sperm transfer
SIN	salpingitis isthmica nodosa
SLE	systemic lupus erythematosus
SPA	sperm penetration assay
STD	sexually transmitted disease
SUZI	subzonal insemination
T_3	triiodothyronine
T_4	thyroxine
TAH	total abdominal hysterectomy
TAT	tray agglutination test
TB	tuberculosis
TESA	testicular sperm aspiration
TESE	testicular sperm extraction
TSH	thyroid stimulating hormone
T-T	tail to tail (sperm) agglutination
TUDOR	transvaginal ultrasound directed oocyte retrieval
UK	United Kingdom
U/S	ultrasound
UTJ	utero-tubal junction
VAP	average path velocity (sperm)
VCL	curvilinear velocity (sperm)
VD	venereal disease
VIN	vulval intra-epithelial neoplasia
VLA	Voluntary Licensing Authority
VSL	straight line velocity (sperm)
WHO	World Health Organisation
ZD	zona drilling
ZIFT	zygote intrafallopian transfer

Appendix 2

Drugs

The following list gives the proprietary names of some of the drugs used in reproductive medicine. It is by no means complete and refers primarily to drugs listed under their generic name in the text. A few proprietary names have been included in the text because of their frequent use and familiarity. Drugs used mainly for hormone replacement therapy or oral contraception, such as ethinyl oestradiol, gestodene, levonorgesterol, mestranol, norgestimate, norgestrel and premarin have not been included.

Generic name	*Proprietary equivalents*
Bromocriptine	Parlodel
Buserelin	Suprecur
	Suprefact
Cyproterone acetate	Androcur
	Cyprostat
Cabergoline	Dostinex
Carbocysteine	Mucodyne
Clomiphene citrate	Clomid
	Serophene
Chorionic gonadotrophin	Gonadotraphon LH
	Pregnyl
	Profasi
Danazol	Danol
Diethyl stilboestrol	Tampovagan
Dydrogesterone	Duphaston
Ethamsylate	Diocynene
Follitrophin α	Gonal-F
Follitrophin β	Puregon
Gestrinone	Dimetriose
Gonadorelin	Fertiral
Goserilin	Zoladex
Human menopausal gonadotrophin	Normegon
Leuprorelin	Prostap SR

Medroxyprogesterone acetate	Depo Provera
	Provera
	Farlutal
Mefenamic acid	Meflam
	Ponstan
Menotrophin	Humegon
	Pergonal
Mesterolone	Pro-Viron
Methotrexate	Maxtrex
Metronidazole	Flagyl
	Zadstat
Mifepristone (RU486)	Mifegyne
Nafarelin	Synarel
Norethisterone	Primolut-N
	Utovlan
Pentoxifylline	Trental
Prednisolone	Deltacortril
Progesterone	Cyclogest
	Gestone
Quinagolide	Norprolac
Tamoxifen	Nolvadex
	Tamofen
Testosterone oenanthate	Primoteston Depot
Testosterone undecanoate	Restandol
Urofollitrophin	Metrodin HP
	Orgafol

Drugs: subsections

Oestrogens: conjugated equine oestrogens, diethyl stilboestrol, ethinyl oestradiol, oestradiol valerate, micronized 17β oestradiol.

Anti-oestrogens: clomiphene citrate, tamoxifen.

Progestogens: dydrogesterone, medroxyprogesterone acetate, norethisterone, progesterone.

Anti-progesterone: mifepristone (RU486).

Androgens: pentoxifylline, testosterone.

Anti-androgens: cyproterone acetate.

Dopamine agonists: bromocriptine, cabergoline, quinagolide.

Gonadotrophins: follitrophin α & β, human chorionic gonadotrophin, human menopausal gonadotrophin, menotrophin, urofollitrophin.

GnRH agonist analogues: buserelin, gonadorelin, goserelin, leuprorelin, nafarelin.

Gonadrotrophin release inhibitors: danazol, gestrinone.